THE CANCER G[

P.O. B[

BEVERLY HILLS

CALIFORNIA – 90213-2832

cancergroup@gmail.com

818.253.4385

WWW.CANCERGROUP.COM

WHAT YOU NEED TO KNOW ABOUT POLYCYTHEMIA VERA

Disclaimer

CancerGroup.com serves only as a clearinghouse for medical and health information and does not directly or indirectly practice medicine. Any information provided by *CancerGroup.com* is intended solely for educating our clients and should not be construed as medical advice or guidance, which should always be obtained from a physician or other licensed health care professional. As such, the client assumes full responsibility for the appropriate use of medical information contained in this book and agrees to hold *CancerGroup.com* and any of its third party providers harmless from any and all claims or actions arising from clients' use or reliance on this guide. Although *CancerGroup.com* makes every reasonable attempt to conduct a thorough search of the published medical literature, the possibility exists that some significant articles may be missed. The statements found throughout have not been evaluated by the Food and Drug Administration. These products are not intended to diagnose, treat, cure, or prevent any disease.

What is Polycythemia Vera?

Polycythemia Vera (PV) or **Primary Polycythemia** is a blood disorder in which bone marrow makes too many red blood cells.

The symptoms of Polycythemia Vera are not visible for many years and it develops very slowly. Lots of people find out about their PV from blood tests done for other reasons.

You may have heard it called PCV, this is incorrect. This is a totally different disease **related to the eye**. Known as Peripheral Polypoidal Choroidal Vasculopathy (PCV).

There are other types of Polycythemia Vera, which we will discuss later in this review.

PV is **NOT** actually "cancer", since the Red Blood Cells that are overproduced do not go on to divide themselves.

Rather, it is a **"myeloproliferative disorder"**, which simply means that too many **NORMAL** Red Blood Cells are being made.

A problem with any myeloproliferative disorder is that the bone marrow loses **"equilibrium"** and does not make necessary cells in the proper ratios.

This impacts all the cells normally produced by the bone marrow.

In Polycythemia vera, the **excess** of red blood cells **increases** the volume of blood and makes it thicker, hence it flows less easily and more slowly through small blood vessels.

This is not good.

To understand PV, we need to discuss what the **normal bone marrow** is and how it functions. Then we will look at the specifics of PV.

Any disease, problem or trouble that G-d gives has a cure. It is basically up to us to find the right person/physician who can channel these cures.

The cure is always available; we just have to know where to look.

In its most simplistic terms, any math question has a correct answer, its' up to us to find it. We may not understand the mathematics behind the problem, but its answer is available.

This formula, which I name the **"Braham Theory of Discovery"**, is correct across every dimension and disease known and even not known to man.

This is how the **"Braham Theory of Discovery"** works in action.

The cure is always available; we just have to know where to look.

What is the Bone Marrow?

The bony skeleton of our body has **two major functions**. The first is to support our frame against the constant pull of gravity, so that we may grow tall instead of flat!

This is primarily done by the hard white **"cortex"** of each bone, which is the outside portion. Inside of most bones is a network of small **"spicules."**

Spicules are tiny spike-like structures (little spines) which are softer than the cortex; the bone is mostly hollow.

These "spicules" of bone are very rich in blood, have special cells gathered upon them which produce new blood, and are called the **"bone marrow"**.

It is easy to visualize this when looking at a large bone from the butcher shop, sawed in half. One will see the hard thick white cortex, over which a thin translucent membrane (**"periosteum"**) is tightly bound.

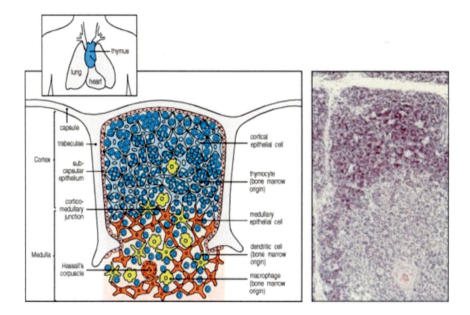

Within the shaft of the bone, the softer marrow will be soaked with blood, and may be scraped out with a knife. This leaves the nerves of the bone in the **Periosteum**, (The Periosteum is a membrane that lines the outer surface of all bones, except at the joints of long bones).

this is the area where the bone "cracks" when broken or invaded by cancer.

There are periodic holes ("fossas") seen in the cortex of the bone where blood vessels penetrate through to nourish the bone and marrow, and carry away newly formed blood from the marrow.

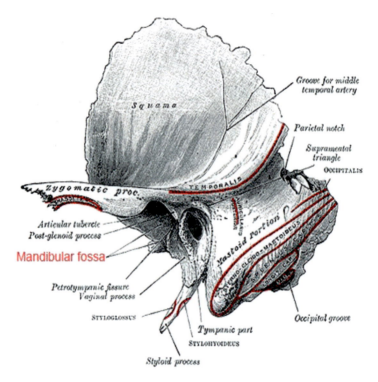

While forming in the womb and through early childhood, the cortex of the bones are made up of **"cartilage"**.

This is a strongly woven but soft connective tissue. Two basic types of bone form, the first being **"long bones"** are seen in the extremities, and the second being **"flat bones"** as found in the skull, hips and vertebrae.

Both types of bones have the inner hollow where the marrow develops. In long bones the cortex encircles the marrow, while in flat bones the cortex is like two "plates" which sandwich the marrow.

While the cortex is initially made of soft cartilage, it is gradually replaced by hard, immature bone.

This is accomplished by a bone forming cell called the **"osteoblast"**, which lays down hard mineral calcium into the cartilage to convert it to bone.

This happens both **within** the cortex, and in the **spicules** of the marrow.

The bone, as first formed in early childhood is **not** as strong as adult bone, so it has to be reformatted by a process, whereby immature bone is re-absorbed through puberty, by cells called **"osteoclasts."**

This is a type of bone cell that removes bone tissue by removing its mineralized matrix and breaking up the organic bone (organic dry weight is 90% collagen).

These osteoclasts return the calcium in the immature bone to the bloodstream. Simultaneously, new **"mature"** bone is layered down in stronger patterns by the **osteoblasts**; which are **mononucleate cells** that are responsible for bone formation. This then will become the permanent bone.

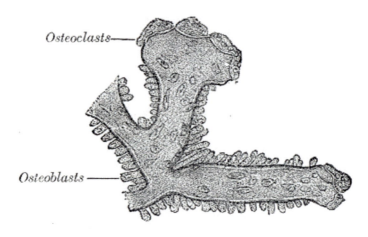

Osteoclasts & osteoblasts of the bone

Mature long bones have **"Haversian Canals"**, these are cylindrical structures that run down the length of the bone to re-enforce it-- much like cement rods.

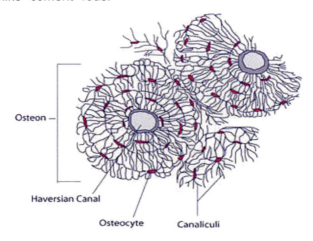

Haversian Canal

These canals also allow blood vessels to travel within their hollow centers, to nourish the bone. Even though mature bone is fully calcified, it still is full of living cells and is subject to infection from germs **("osteomyelitis")** or dying **("Avascular necrosis")**.

The symptoms of these problems are usually severe, demanding prompt expert attention.

Long bones are described by their shaft **("diaphysis")**, area near their growing ends **("metaphysis")** and the actual ends **("epiphysis")**.

Marrow tends to be most plentiful in **"proximal extremities"** -- long bones nearer to the center of the body (e.g. thigh and upper arm), with relatively less in the **"distal extremities"** (e.g. fingers and toes).

The marrow actually recedes closer to the center of the body as we age. Flat bones are described by their aspect closes to the skin **("outer table")**, "middle marrow", and the portion deepest in the body **("inner table")**.

They can have very irregular shapes, as seen in the vertebrae and pubic bones, and they are generally rich in marrow. One can puncture the hard cortex with a special boring needle and suck out the soft marrow inside the bone-- this is called a **"bone marrow aspiration"**.

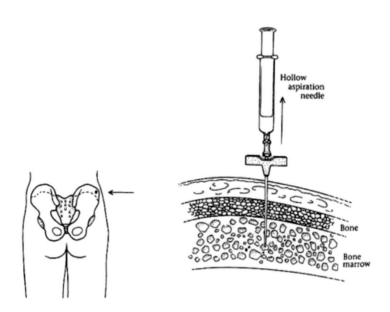

Bone Marrow Aspiration

It is usually performed on bones with a thin cortex, lots of marrow, and near the skin surface. The site most commonly chosen to aspirate bone marrow for testing or transplant are the paired **"iliac wings"**-- the flaring hip bones at the belt line level, above each buttock. An aspiration may be done from one side or both, depending upon the circumstance.

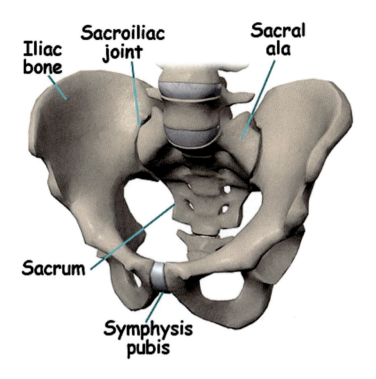

iliac wings

For understanding bone marrow transplant, we must understand how the normal marrow works. The marrow is a wonderful cell-synthesizing laboratory, which repopulates the blood with crucial cells that are essential to life.

Normally the marrow is producing new cells by the billions every day, never stopping until the person dies.

This contrasts strongly with most other body systems, which make the majority of their cells during womb life and childhood, **slowly drastically** in the mature adult.

Furthermore, the marrow can be activated in response to stress, such as bleeding, infection, or shock, to go into high gear and crank out blood cells quickly.

If the marrow fails, we expect rapid, progressive problems with **infections,** poor **blood clotting**, and **anemia** (in that order). We will now examine the individual cells in the marrow that go on to serve these purposes.

The bony spicules in the marrow serve to support it, giving it a lose network structure which serves as an expansion base and surface area for new cells to form.

The spicules were themselves formed by the osteoblasts, as mentioned. Aside from the bony spicules, and fat and connective tissue which may infiltrate the marrow, all cells developing in the marrow arise from a single type of **"precursor"** cell.

This precursor is called the **"Pluripotential Stem Cell"** or **"Stem Cell"** for short.

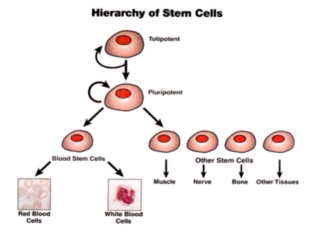

These Stem Cells can, and do, develop into every known type of blood cell-- a process known as cell **"differentiation"**.

Firstly, the Stem Cells divide to produce other Stem Cells. Then, they divide into 2 major lines-- the **"Lymphoid"** and **"Myeloid"** lines. The "Lymphoid" cells go on to mature into crucial White Blood Cells called **"Lymphocytes"**.

These will be further described later, since they are critical to proper immune system activity in preventing infections.

The **"Myeloid"** cells differentiate into 4 other major White Blood Cell groups-- the **"Neutrophils"**, **"Basophils"**, **"Monocytes"** and **"Eosinophils"**. **Erythrocytes** also come from the Myeloid Line.

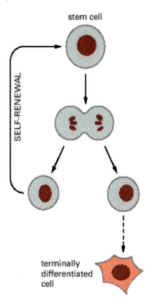

The definition of a stem cell

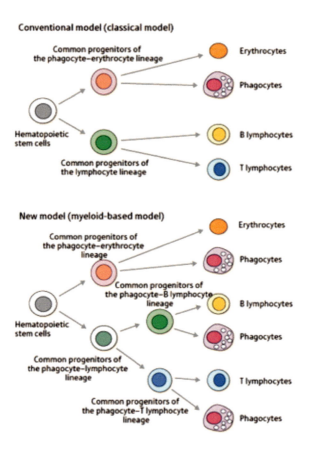

Erythrocytes is another name for **Red Blood Cells**. Polycythemia Vera will be seen to be a disorder of the Myeloid Cell Line maturation.

Each of these cell types are standardly found when examining a **"smear"** of whole blood or the bone marrow.

This smear is called a **"differential"**, it gives the type and number of White Blood Cells and Red Blood Cells seen.

Regarding White Blood Cells:

1) Lymphocytes 60% in children, 30% in adults-- especially increase with viruses.

2) Neutrophils 30% in children, 60% in adults-- especially increase with bacteria.

3) Monocytes-- about 5-10% in children or adults, increase with viral infections.

4) Eosinophils -- 2-5% in children & adults, increased by allergies or parasites.

5) Basophils-- 1% in children & adults, do not commonly increase with infection.

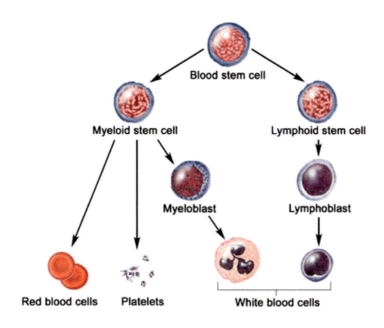

Blood cell development. A blood stem cell goes through several steps to become a red blood cell, platelet, or white blood cell.

Not only do the relative percentages of certain White Blood Cells increase with infections or inflammation, but the total number (per milliliter of whole blood) usually do also.

For instance, a normal White Blood Cell count is 4,000 to 10,000 per milliliter, with infections this may increase by several thousand-- or even tens of thousands.

An exception is if the White Blood Cells are being **"consumed"** by the invading germ-- leading to an initial decrease in the number of circulating cells. Another reason that White Blood Cells may be drastically increased is when a cancer of White Blood Cells occurs-- called a **"leukemia"**. However, even though the absolute number of [cancerous] White Cells may be increased (sometimes over 100,000 per milliliter) they are ineffective at fighting infection and actually retard immune system functioning.

White Blood Cells tend to live between 8 hours and 20 years (depending upon the subtype). The majority of important Neutrophils (also called **"Granulocytes"**) are short lived, just 12 to 36 hours, and so they must be continuously replenished by the bone marrow.

If the marrow **"Fails"** and produces no cells at all (**"pancytopenia"**) then **infection** will be the **1st sign**.

If accompanied by a fever (as is common), the condition of insuffient Granulocytes is called **"Febrile Neutropenia"** and is usually fatal if not quickly addressed with multiple antibiotics **("triple therapy")**.

As will be seen, febrile Neutropenia is a known, and commonly deadly complication of aggressive therapy for PV.

Thankfully we have better tools to deal with it now than ever before.

To form the **Red Blood Cells** and **Platelets**, the Myeloid line further splits into two other crucial types of blood component forming cells-- the **"Erythroblasts"** and the **"Megakaryocytes"**. The Erythroblasts go on to differentiate into the **"Erythocytes"**-- they are the **"Red Blood Cells"**.

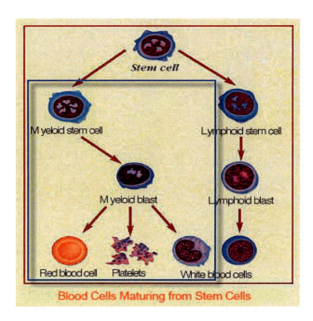

Blood Cells Maturing from Stem Cells

These circulate within the bloodstream, carrying fresh oxygen (from the lungs) to the body cells.

They also collect and transport the waste product "carbon dioxide" (produced by metabolizing sugar) from the body cells back to the lungs to be breathed out.

The actual substance within the Red Blood Cells which transports oxygen is called **"Hemoglobin"**, and contains Iron and makes the whole blood red in color. Normally, Red Blood Cell production is stimulated by a protein called **"Erythropoetin"** produced by the kidneys.

As will be seen, this protein has been artificially synthesized and is very helpful in stimulating new Red Blood Cell production if there are Stem Cells present.

When there are insufficient Red Blood Cells circulating, the **"oxygen tension"** of the blood will decrease, and the body is in danger of suffocating.

There are typically 11 to 16 grams of Hemoglobin per 100 milliliters ("deciliter") of blood, with men having a higher amount than women.

If the Hemoglobin is too low, this is called **"anemia"**. Various anemias have different causes **("etiologies")**.

Examples include too little Iron intake (**"Iron Deficiency Anemia"**) where the Red Blood Cells look small **("microcytic")**, pale and washed out, and Folate or Vitamin B-12 Deficiency where they are too large **("megaloblastic")**.

Also, of course, an anemia can arise as a result of failure of the bone marrow to produce blood cells **("aplastic anemia")**. This can result from a cancer invading the bone marrow, getting too much toxic chemotherapy or irradiation which kills the marrow, or even as a birth defect ("Blackfan's anemia").

Whatever the cause, too few oxygen carrying Red Blood Cells results in patients being pale, weak, dizzy and fatigued. Patients will usually be get a **"transfusion"** of Packed Red Blood Cells when their Hemoglobin falls below 8.0 grams or when they start getting **"symptomatic"**-- with shortness of breath, palpitations, or severe weakness and dizzyness.

Once **"Packed Unit"** of Red Cells **("RBC's)** usually **raises** the hemoglobin by about 1.0 gram, so several **"units"** are commonly necessary.

Normally Red Blood Cells live ~120 days, so if the Bone Marrow FAILS completely infection will be seen prior to Red Cell anemia.

The final important Myeloid cell line are the **"Megakaryocytes"**, giant cells which produce **"Platelets"** essential to blood clotting.

Platelets are not actual cells (as White cells and Red cells are) but "fragments" of membranous material. Platelets contain special enzymes which become activated on contact with air.

In conjunction with an elaborate "cascade" of enzymatic reactions from "clotting factors" produced by the liver, as well as from "substrate" proteins from injured blood vessels, platelets form clots.

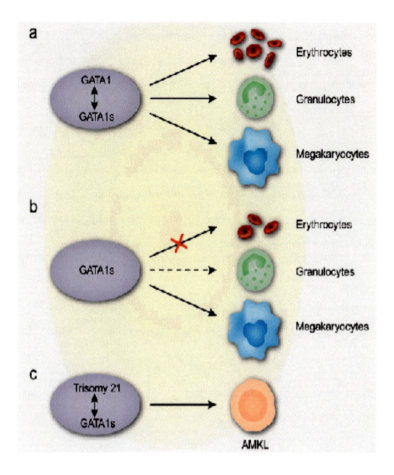

Normally, the platelet count is between 150,000 and 400,000 per milliliter of whole blood.

Low platelets are seen with many leukemias, with intense chemotherapy, and with a failing bone marrow.

A low platelet count is called **"thrombocytopenia"** and is a serious medical concern. The patient with low platelets will show easy bruising (**"echymosis"**), and a prolonged **"bleeding time"** if injured.

Platelet counts below 50,000 are considered worrisome, and below 20,000 demand a **"transfusion"** of platelets. This is owing to the high risk of spontaneous internal bleeding **("hemorrhage")** with such low platelet counts.

Interestingly, the common drug aspirin irreversibly damages the enzymatic clotting ability of platelets, and raises bleeding time.

This is why aspirin is **discouraged** ("contraindicated") in late pregnancy and prior to major surgery or at the dentist.

Normally platelets "live" (they are not really alive) for 10 days after being released by the Megakaryocytes into the bone marrow, and carried into the bloodstream.

A transfused **"unit"** of platelets typically raises the Platelet Count by 10,000, so many units are often necessary.

To complicate matters, the body's immune system can become sensitized to, and destroy, transfused platelets as **"foreign bodies"**.

The more transfusions a person has had, the greater the risk for this immune response. If the person can produce their own platelets, the body's immune system will generally not destroy them.

This is far preferable to transfusions which at best last a couple weeks. Again, the increasing order of longevity for blood cells is **White Cells, Platelets**, and then **Red Blood Cells**.

Thus, if a person has total failure of the bone marrow, the **first** sign (within days) will be infection **due to low White Count**, the **second** (within weeks) is easy bruising due to low Platelets, and the **third** (within months) is Anemia due to low Red Cells count.

In practice, infection and internal bleeding are lethal before anemia becomes a noticeable **("clinical")** problem. Nonetheless, transfusions are RBC's are frequently necessary to combat the anemia of partial bone marrow failure.

In Polycythemia Vera an inordinately large number of Red Blood Cells are produced, but often at the expense of fewer normal White Blood Cells and Platelets.

You can see that the Bone Marrow comprises a very dynamic system for new blood cell production, without which the body will fail rapidly.

What is the Difference between Bone Marrow and Circulating Blood?

The Bone Marrow is the **"factory"** where new cells are manufactured, but most move out into systemic circulation.

The marrow tends to be densely **"packed"** with cells, while in the whole blood they are diluted by the blood serum.

Commonly, less **"mature"** forms of cells are found in the marrow than in circulating blood.

For instance, fledgling Red Blood Cells formed in the marrow (from erythroblasts) still have a **nucleus**, and are called **"reticulocytes"** which are immature red blood cells, typically composing about 1% of the red cells in the human body.

Once they migrate out into the circulation, they **lose** their nucleus to become the familial disk-shaped Red Blood Cells.

When we find a high number of reticulocytes in the circulating blood, this suggests that **new Red Cells** are being formed very rapidly in response to bleeding.

On the other hand, finding too few in the bone marrow presages failure of production and eventual anemia.

To properly diagnose persistent **("refractory")** anemias, we need to get a **sample of bone marrow** to see what is going on there.

These anemias can be the harbingers of leukemias, since Red Cell production usually **goes down** as abnormal White Blood Cell production **goes up**.

The White Blood Cells formed in the marrow similarly tend to be less mature, and when they go into the circulating blood they may cling ("adhere") onto blood vessel walls or go into lymph nodes. There they mature as they are exposed to foreign proteins **("antigens")**. They also subdivide into their particular classes of lymphocytes, such as "**B**" and "**T**" cells, after they are released from the marrow.

Stress to the body (i.e. from trauma or infection) releases stress hormones (i.e. cortisol) which **"demarginate"** White Blood Cells out of their sanctuary areas, and quickly raise their level in the circulation.

This explains how the circulating **WBC** count can go up so rapidly, before the bone marrow has time to **"respond"** to the stress.

Platelets are usually released into the circulation as soon as they are formed. They are not alive and do not require maturation time.

However, they will go up quickly with shock or stress, as a result of the **"Megakaryocytes"** in the bone marrow releasing young platelets.

The blood vessels to the marrow are "two way streets"; they take new cells out and return established cells (from the circulation) back in.

This is how the bone marrow gets nourishment and oxygen.

However, this process can transmit infection or cancer cells into the bone marrow. The bone marrow is a delicate "organ" which can easily become damaged.

When damage occurs, then problems such as White Blood Cell cancers (e.g. leukemia, lymphoma), Red Cell Cancers ("erythroleukemia") and Myeloproliferative Disorders like Polycythemia Vera can result.

What are the Different Types of Polycythemia?

The term "polycythemia" itself means that there are too many cells, but it is not specific as to the reason for this.

The first type is called **"Absolute Polycythemia"**, and is seen in all newborns. In fetal life, much less oxygen is delivered through the umbilical cord than will be obtained at birth when the lungs start functioning.

Since Red Blood Cells carry the oxygen, many more of them are needed in fetal life-- and thus newborns have **"high"** hematocrits (over 50% of their blood volume is RBC's).

The excess RBC's are rapidly destroyed in the first few weeks after birth; the inability of the immature liver to handle the breakdown products of these RBC's accounts for the newborn jaundice commonly seen.

Thus, technically, all newborns suffer from relative "polycythemia".

A **"Relative Polycythemia"** occurs when there is a dramatic loss of blood fluid volume without losing RBC's-- as occurs with severe dehydration.

In Relative Polycythemia, there is not an inordinate number of RBC's being produced-- instead the concentration of them is too high owing to loss of diluting blood fluid.

A **"Compensatory Polycythemia"** means that more RBC's are required due to low oxygen delivery to the body tissues. For example, if people live at very high elevations, where the air is rarified, they will need relatively more RBC's to latch onto the available oxygen.

Their blood counts will slowly normalize if they return to live at low altitudes. Also, if patients suffer from lung diseases like emphysema that interfere with diffusion of oxygen between the lungs and RBC's, then more RBC's will be needed to absorb what oxygen does get through.

"Stress Polycythemia" is a condition affecting mostly white, middle aged, mildly obese men who are physically active and anxiety prone-- but in contrast to Polycythemia Vera, only RBC's are elevated-- not other blood cells.

Lastly, **"Polycythemia Vera"** is a myeloproferative disorder of unknown origin where **ALL BLOOD CELL COMPONENTS ARE INCREASED.**

Thus we expect to see an increase in concentration of White Blood Cells and Platelets in Polycythemia Vera, as well as RBC's.

The thick Red Cell mass makes the blood more viscous and sluggish-- problems seen in all cases severe polycythemia. The increase in RBC's is the most significant factor in Polycythemia Vera-- since they contribute the most viscosity to the circulating blood.

The increase in Platelets and White cells will be further discussed.

What Causes Polycythemia Vera?

The cause of Polycythemia Vera **is unknown**-- however various **"risk factors"** for contracting the disease have been identified.

These are recognized by studying groups of patients for common elements in their histories. Factors increasing risk are:

1) Male Gender-- PV is slightly more common in men. The reasons for this may be due to a higher baseline hemoglobin in males, generally 14.0 -16.0 as opposed to females who normally run 12.0 - 14.0. Men make more red cells.

2) White Race-- The disease is uncommon in Blacks and Asians. It is most common in American and European caucasians.

3) Age-- The disease is most common to develop in late **middle age**, the average patient is 55 years old. The disease is exceeding **rare in children**.

4) Jewish Extraction-- PV is found with increased frequency in Jews and other peoples of Mediterranean family origin.

5) Chromosome Damage-- All myelodysplastic syndromes, and cancers for that matter, are thought due to critical genetic damage within a particular cell.

Many things can cause genetic damage presaging disease, including intake of chemicals, radiation exposure, or inborn (**inherited**) gene problems.

We have yet to identify every initiating sequence of gene damage that leads to PV. At the present time, abnormal chromosome patterns are seen in 15% of untreated patients with PV and 30% of treated patients.

The abnormal structures most commonly involve a duplication of the long arm of Chromosome #1, deletion of the long arm of Chromosome #20, and bone marrow cells with duplication of chromosomes # 8 and 9. If PV proceeds to leukemia (see below) then 85% of these patients can be shown to have had abnormal Chromosome patterns.

Within the "leukemic phase" of PV that some patients develop, loss of material from **Chromosome #7** is seen in 20% and from the long arm of **Chromosome #5** is seen in 40%.

These changes may be due to prior treatment.

With the ongoing Human Genome Project, we expect to define more clearly the genes involved.

6) Family Disposition-- In spite of the factors above, paradoxically PV is rarely found in more than one member of a single family at a time. Thus other family members have little reason to be concerned about **"inheriting"** the disease.

How Common Is Polycythemia Vera?

It is difficult to say exactly how common PV is, since many patients **"smolder"** with it for years without coming to medical attention.

Since many of these patients are elderly, they end up succumbing to some other (**"comorbid"**) medical condition like a heart attack or stroke.

A reasonable estimate of the number of any people in the U.S.A affected at any given time (**"point prevalence"**) is **40,000** patients.

Worldwide the disease follows the proportion of aging caucasians. The disease appears to be more common now with the general aging of the population.

What are the Signs and Symptoms of Polycythemia Vera?

A **"sign"** is something that **can be measured**, such as fever or spleen size.

A **"symptom"** is something felt by the patient, such as fatigue or headache. Common manifestations of Polycythemia Vera include:

1) Plethora-- this means increased redness (" ruddiness") of the body, especially noticeable in the face, neck and hands and feet. Normally we see plethora in newborns, who have temporarily high hematocrits. The redness is from increase in RBC's flowing through these areas. The plethora will get more severe with rising hematocrit-- indicating worsening disease. Conversely, the plethora will diminish with effective therapy.

2) Headache is of pounding nature and thought due to both a decrease in the amount of blood permeating the brain (**"cerebral perfusion"**) and an increase in the viscosity of the blood. Similarly, headache is seen when patients have high blood pressure, since the blood vessels supplying the brain constrict and patients end up with less blood perfusing the brain.

3) Dizziness and Vertigo-- Dizziness is a feeling a unsteadiness as though one might faint, and vertigo is a sensation of the room spinning around. These are both caused by decreased blood flow throughout the brain. A **"rushing"** sensation in the ears and a sensation of "fullness" in the head are also common. Outright fainting spells ("syncope") may occur with very **"viscous blood"** (thickened).

4) Visual Changes-- These also result from decreased blood flow to the visual nerves (cranial nerve II) and the part of the brain that interprets vision (occipital lobe). Changes include visualizing starts or **"fortification"** structures that are not there, double vision, or blurred vision.

5) Blood Clotting-- Over 35% of patients have an episode of abnormal bleeding ("hemorrhage") or premature blood clotting (**"thrombosis"**) during the disease. If spontaneous bleeding occurs, it is commonest from the nose or a peptic ulcer.

There can also be easy bruising in the muscles and joints. Too rapid clotting of blood can result in heart attack, stroke, or clots in the lungs (pulmonary embolism).

Whenever the blood is too thick and viscous, the changes of spontaneous clotting are increased. There is also acceleration of **"hardening of the arteries"**-- that is calcified plaques forming within the interior (**"lumen"**) of arteries, in those with PCV. This simultaneously contributes to higher risk of heart attack or stroke.

6) Itching ("Pruritis") is common in PCV patients and is particularly severe after bathing. It may be so bad as to be disabling. Easy formation of welts ("**uticaria**") may also be observed.

7) Gout and Kidney Stones are the result of too much uric acid building up in the tissues and kidneys. The excess of uric acid is due to the body's attempt to breakdown the excessive number of blood cells being produced.

With chronic high uric acid, the kidneys eventually may start to fail (uric acid nephropathy).

Fortunately there are medications available that gets rid of excess uric acid in blood plasma called **allopurinal.**

8) Spleen Enlargement is due to trapping Red Blood Cells and Platelets by this organ.

The spleen is located in the left upper abdomen and normally is above the bottom rib on the left side.

With enlargement ("**splenomegaly**") it can grow to huge sizes, giving a feeling of bloating in the abdomen, increasing belt-size, and interfering with eating and digestion.

The capsule surrounding the spleen contains its nerves, and so pain may be felt in the left upper abdomen with an enlargement of the spleen.

Occasionally the enlargement may be so dramatic that it is advisable to remove the spleen surgically ("**splenectomy**"), or possibly shrink it using low dose radiation therapy.

9) Leukemia-- PV predisposes to leukemia, but it occurs in just 2% of those patients getting no treatment except bloodletting ("phlebotomy"-- see below).

Up to 15% of patients getting treated with specific drugs may get leukemia.

How is Polycythemia Vera Diagnosed?

Many patients with PV are incidentally diagnosed when they come in to get a blood test for some other purpose, such as prior to an elective surgery.

It is common to see patients without the full "**clinical spectrum**" of the disease-- that is mild manifestations. If a patients "**presents**" appearing **plethoric** (ruddy), has an enlarged spleen, shows increases in all blood cell elements on their **Complete Blood Count** ("CBC") and has no obvious heart or lung disease, then the diagnosis is straightforward.

However, in many patients increased hemoglobin or hematocrit is discovered at routine laboratory evaluation, and then it is important that the diagnosis of PV be properly confirmed.

The **first step** is to rule-out that the increase in hemoglobin concentration is due to dehydration called ("**relative polycythemia**"), which is an apparent **rise** of the erythrocyte level in the blood.

Or it is due to heart or lung disease that is preventing **proper oxygen concentrations** from getting to the body tissues.

There are tests to measure the actual blood cell mass, to determine whether the hormone erythropoetin is increased, and to look for kidney tumors ("**hypernephroma**") that might be increasing Red Blood Cell mass.

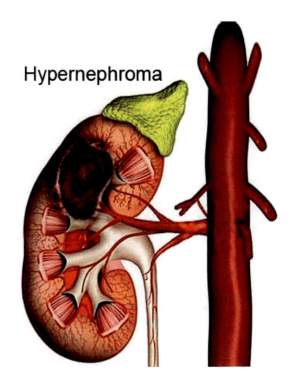

Hypernephroma

The tests to diagnose PV, from most common to most complex, are as follows:

a) Red Blood Cell Count-- the Red Blood Cells, or "RBC's" carry oxygen to body cells and take carbon dioxide away from them.

RBC's are made in the bone marrow by the **"erythroid"** precursor cells; they are stimulated by lack of oxygen and by the kidney hormone erythropeitin.

Chronic bleeding, malnutrition, invasion of the bone marrow by cancer, chemotherapy, and radiation can all lower the RBC count, and then the patient is **"anemic"** and appears pale and fatigued.

Very low counts can cause heart attacks for lack of oxygen to the heart muscle. Red Cells commonly live 120 days in the circulation, and if they are low they can be transfused as **"Packed RBC's"**.

A normal RBC count is between **4** and **6 million per milliliter** of whole blood. In PV patients, the character of the RBC's may be pale and washed out looking due to a decrease in available iron (see below).

b) Hematocrit also refers to the Red Blood Cells, this indicator shows what the percent volume of the whole blood is that they occupy.

That is, if we take a tube of whole blood, and call the top level 100%, we can "spin it down" in a centrifuge and the RBC's will compact on the bottom, leaving the clear fluid serum floating on top.

The percent of volume that these packed cells occupy is called the **hematocrit**.

In Polycythemia Vera and dehydration, there are too many RBC's in the blood for the available serum, and the hematocrit is high.

In anemic conditions, there are **too few** RBC's and the hematocrit is dangerously low.

A normal hematocrit level is between 40% and 50%; it is **higher** in men than women. In PV the hematocrit (**packed cell volume**) is commonly in the 60% range.

c) **Hemoglobin** is the **iron** containing protein which actually carries oxygen in the RBC's and gives the blood its red color.

It is low if the patient has too few RBC's or is deficient in iron or **vitamin B12** or **Folic acid** necessary to make RBC's.

We use the hemoglobin value to decide when to transfuse patients. In general, each **"Unit"** of Packed RBC's raises the hemoglobin value by 2 points.

Normal hemoglobin is ~12 grams per deciliter in women and 14 grams per deciliter in men.

Below 8 grams, patients start showing severe symptoms of anemia. In patients with PCV, the hemoglobin is commonly about 18 grams per deciliter but can be quickly reduced by bleeding the patient (discussed ahead).

d) **Red Blood Cell Indices** include **Mean Cell Volume** or **MCV** which says how big the average RBC is. RBC's will be too small and look washed out if the patient is iron deficient, this commonly occurs with chronic bleeds.

This is called a **"microcytic anemia"**. Conversely, they will be too big if the patient is deficient in vitamin B12 or Folate.

This is called a **"megaloblastic anemia"**, Normal MCV is between 85 and 95.

Mean Corpuscle Hemoglobin Concentration or **MCHC** is gotten by dividing the hemoglobin by the number of RBC's to figure how much hemoglobin is in each one, so it tells how well the RBC's are packaging hemoglobin.

Mean Corpuscle Hemoglobin of MCH tells the same thing but uses the hematocrit instead of the hemoglobin to divide into.

All of these tests tell how normal in size and color the RBC's are. In PV, we often see an iron deficiency anemia with a smaller RBC size than normal (**"microcytosis"**). There may be a variety of shades of red to the RBC's (**"polychromasia"**).

e) **White Blood Cell Count** or **WBC's** is a very important indicator of how well the bone marrow is **making new White Cells.**

These will be lowered by Chemotherapy that **suppresses** the bone marrow, by **cancer** invading bone marrow, by Radiation Therapy certain leukemias, rapid infections that are gobbling up the existing WBC's, and chronic steroid use.

Conversely, WBC's will be very high in **specific Chronic Leukemias** where lots of abnormal ones are being manufactured (they don't work to combat infection) and with infections when the bone marrow is capable of generating WBC's to fight germs.

There are **sub-types** of WBC's which will be discussed below under "**Differential**".

A normal total WBC count is between 3 and 10 thousand per milliliter. In PV, we often see an elevated WBC count of 15,000 - 25,000 per milliliter, it sometimes gets as **high as 60,000** without indicating infection. Remember that in PV, **all** the blood cell elements are **increased.**

f) Platelet Count is a measure of fragments put out by giant "**megakaryocyte**" cells in the bone marrow; these fragments are not individually "alive" but help form blood clots.

Low platelets is called **"thrombocytopenia"** and is caused by chemotherapy that **suppresses** the bone marrow, antibodies formed by WBC's against our own platelets in "auto-immune diseases" like **Idiopathic Thrombocytopenic Purpura** (ITP), and certain leukemias that interfere with production of platelets.

ITP is a bleeding condition in which the blood doesn't clot as it should.

The platelets will also be lowered by **"consumptive coagulopathies"** that are forming lots of clots in the bloodstream and using up all of the available platelets, like DIC.

When they are too **low** (below 100 Thousand) then little purple bumps called **"purpura"** form on the skin.

If the platelets are extremely low (less than 20 Thousand) then the risk is very high for spontaneous internal bleeding.

When platelets are too **high** it is called **"thrombocytosis"** as this is seen with some infections or leukemias of platelet forming megakaryocytes.

Then the risk for spontaneous blood clots increases. Normal platelet counts are 200 to 500 thousand ("200 to 500 K") per milliliter of whole blood.

In PV the platelet count is usually about 500,000 and perhaps as high as 1 million per milliliter.

g) Reticulocytes are **immature** RBC's that still **have** their nucleus, they normally lose this as they move from the bone marrow to circulating blood.

They may be ordered separately from the CBC or as part of it.

They show that new RBCs are capable of being formed in the bone marrow, and normally go up with acute bleeding.

The patient is "reticking" if the reticulocyte count is over 2.0%. In PV we expect a relatively **high number** of reticulocytes owing to the large number of new RBC's being produced.

h) Sedimentation Rate - or also known as erythrocyte sedimentation rate (**ESR**), also called a sedimentation rate or **Biernacki Reaction,** means basically that a sample tube of whole blood is shaken up and the time it takes for the blood cells to settle toward the bottom is measured.

The sedimentation rate is checked over 60 minutes and the normal rate is 10 - 30 millimeters per first hour as measured in a calibrated tube.

It the **"sedrate"** is **higher**, it is a non-specific but important finding. It can mean any sort of inflammation, from **Temporal Arteritis** to **bone infections** to **rheumatoid arthritis**.

It is thus a **"non specific indicator"** of something going on, but it doesn't indicate what.

If it is high, it gives reason to order further tests to determine the cause. In general **"sedrates"** are normally higher in women than men. In PCV, the sedimentation rate is often very low (0 - 3 mm/hr) owing to the viscosity of the blood.

i) Differential means a **visual smear** of the blood cells stained with **Wright's dye** that highlights the cells for microscopic examination.

They are stained a deep purple and counted manually by the Laboratory Technologist. Many subtle details can be told by an experienced microscopist.

The most basic thing to see is the types of cells present and their shape (**"morphology"**). The White Blood Cells, Red Blood

Cells and Platelets can all be visualized as to the number and appearance:

1) White Blood Cells or "**WBC's**" are counted within a small field to 100, and the number of each type is tallied.

The **basic types** of circulating WBC's are:

A) Lymphocytes are relatively small, round, blue staining cells that help fight all sorts of infections. They are plentiful and especially increase with viral infections (or other non-malignant "**leukemoid reaction**" causes) and with lymphoctytic leukemias, notably ALL and CLL.

They normally number about 4000 (but range considerably) per milliliter and comprise 30 - 60% of WBC's depending upon age; children have proportionately more.

The lymphocytes have life-spans of days to decades depending upon subtype, and carry the immune instructions from vaccinations and previous infections.

In PV we expect an increase in all subtypes of WBC's, including lymphocytes.

B) Neutrophils are **large cells** with small "**granules**" in them;

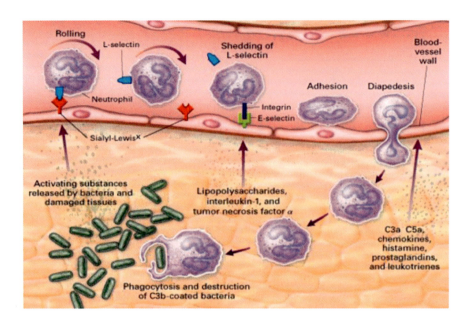

they appear speckled under the microscope and are called **"granulocytes"**.

They are the primary defense against bacterial infections, without granulocytes we are at risk for overwhelming infection of the normally sterile blood, called **"bacteremia"**.

This quickly leads to poisoning of the blood by the bacterial waste products, **"septicemia"**, which is rapidly fatal if unsuccessfully treated.

Neutrophils actually identify and eat (**"phagocytize"**) bacteria, and

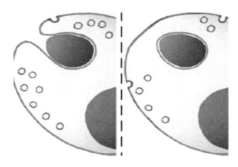

are thus so important that they are the WBC's we transfuse for low White Count (called **"leucopenic"**) patients.

When they are increased markedly, it generally means either overwhelming infection the body has not had a chance to respond too, a large infection that is being responded to, or myelogenous leukemia like AML or CML.

Normally the total Neutrophil count is over 2000 per milliliter of blood, and they represent 30 - 60% of WBC's depending on age.

We get worried when the neutrophil count is **under** 1000, and especially **below** 500, called **"neutropenia"**. If a fever develops, patients need **immediate triple type intravenous antibiotics** for **"febrile neutropenia"**, and you will be hospitalized.

The nuclei (center portion) of neutrophils seems to expand and show more points sticking out (**"hypersegmented"**) during acute infections.

Neutrophils often live for only 12 - 24 hours in the bloodstream!

In advanced PV, the marrow may **"burn out"** (become "fibrotic") and then less WBC's than normal are produced-- this can predispose to infections.

C) Monocytes look like large lymphocytes and have no granules.

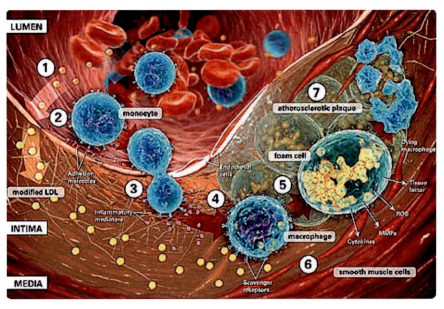

They are important in the detection of germs, as part of the **"monocyte-macrophage"** system.

The macrophages consume invading bacteria after identification, much like neutrophils above.

Monocytes are **increased** with mononucleiosis, ("**kissing disease**"), some other viral infections and rare monocytic leukemia.

The normally represent less than 10% of the circulating blood cells.

D) Eosinophils are also larger than lymphocytes and have red-staining granules floating in their fluid portion ("cytoplasm").

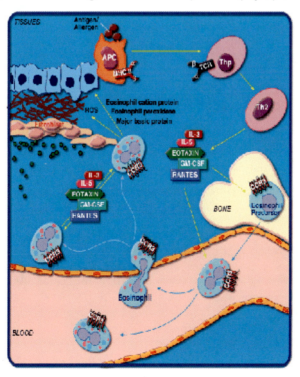

They are important against parasites, protozoa and unusual foreign substances (like wood).

When the number of eosinophils increases it is termed **"eosinophilia"**.

Eosinophils will commonly increase with worm infections, allergies, and rare leukemias arising from them.

They normally represent less than 8% of the circulating blood cells.

E) **Basophils** are large cells with blue staining granules, so are "granuloctyes". They have general immune functions at helping recognize and destroy germs.

Lots of Basophils is called **"basophilia"** and is seen in rare infections or even rarer leukemias arising from basophils.

Normally they comprise just 1 - 2 % of the circulating blood. In PV an increase in the absolute basophil count to about 100 per milliliter is seen in 70% of patients.

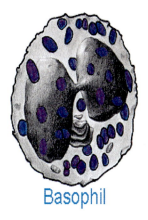
Basophil

F) Blasts are newly minted WBC's that are obviously immature and are being pushed out very quickly by the bone marrow.

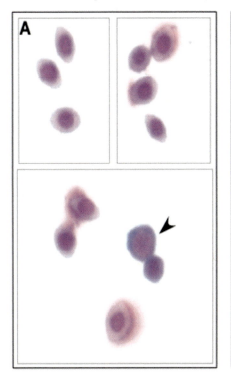
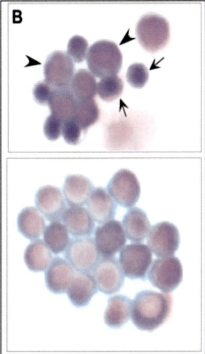

Having blasts shows either a severe infection that the body is responding to, or a leukemic crises ("**blast crises**") where billions of useless blasts are being churned out of the marrow.

We can often distinguish acute from chronic leukemia based upon the blasts.

Various **"smoldering leukemias"** will show a low amount (i.e. <3%) of blasts, and then lots of blasts (ie. >30%) when they **"transform"** into acute leukemia.

Between 2% and 15% of PCV patients will have an eventual transition to an acute leukemia, and a high blast count in the circulating blood may show this.

2) **Red Blood Cells** or "RBC's" are examined as to their character, shape and size during the differential.

Anemia will be obvious by the relative lack of RBCs and the basic subtype can be determined. Lack of iron makes for poor **hemoglobin synthesis**, and so the RBC's are small and washed-out appearing, that is a **"microcytic anemia"**.

This is the most common type in chronic bleeding patients. Poor intake of vitamins B12 and Folate lead to a giant red blood cells, that is a **"megaloblastic anemia"**.

In PV vitamin B-12 levels vary and are increased in about 30% of patients. Chronic disease often leads to anemia with relatively normal sized RBC's, this is called **"normocytic anemia"** or "anemia of chronic disease".

If the red blood cells have nuclei, they are called **"reticulocytes"** and a high count shows that they are being (too) rapidly produced **"reticulocytosis"**.

Sickling of the RBC's makes the diagnosis for sickle cell disease, and lots of other changes in **"morphology"** are witnessed.

If the RBC's have an abnormal array of shapes, it is called **"poikilocytosis"**, and if they vary in size it is called **"anisocytosis"**.

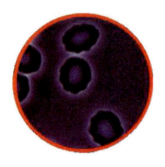

Poikilocytosis

Various rare genetic causes of anemia, like **"thallasemia"** can lead to all sorts of bizarre RBC shapes, like teardrops (**"dacrocytosis"**) or lots of broken up "helmet" and "burr" cells.

Being forced out a bone marrow crowded with cells can produce bizarre shapes, this can indicate a **"myeloproliferative disorder"** where bone marrow gets stuffed with abnormal cells.

Conversely, if the marrow gets "burned out" (**"fibrotic"**) and no longer produces many viable blood cells, the RBC's will have abnormal morphology.

Spleen problems and infections can cause the RBC's to stack like coins, this is the **"Rouleaux sign"**.

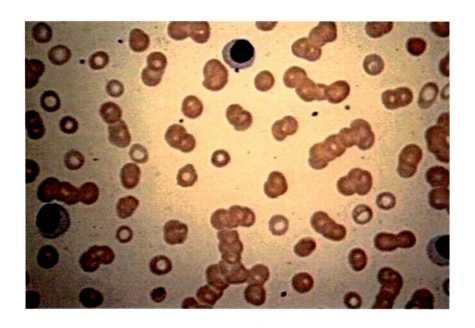

Rouleaux sign

RBC's with rings around them in the bone marrow (**"ringed sideroblasts"**) show lead or other heavy metal poisoning.

Large increase in RBC's is "erythocytosis"; as with Polycythemia Vera.

A common treatment for this is bleeding the patient! It can also show an **"erytho-leukemia"**, since the RBC's and WBC's (excluding the lymphocytes) arise from a common **"precursor"** cell in the bone marrow-- so leukemias can arise as an apparent cross between them!).

In general bizarre patterns of RBC's are called **"dyscrasias"** and may indicate serious diseases.

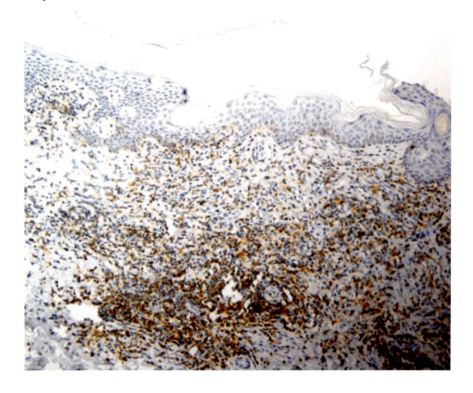

Dyscrasias

3) Platelets-- the number and appearance of the Platelets, discussed previously, is also visually confirmed on the Differential.

In some leukemia patients with swollen spleens (**"spleenomegaly"**), the platelets are "trapped" in there, they show low in the circulating blood, even while the marrow is producing them.

In these patients removing or irradiation the spleen often raises platelet counts. Platelets live an average of 10 days in the circulation.

When platelets are being **transfused**, each "unit" raises the platelet count by about 10K.

However, if the patient has been **"sensitized"** by prior platelet transfusions, their immune system may destroy them very quickly, and daily transfusions may be needed.

In PV the platelets may function poorly, even though there are many of them, leading to easy bleeding (**"bleeding diathesis"**) and hemorrhage.

Alternately, they may clot within the blood vessels (**"intravascularly"**) causing heart attack or stroke.

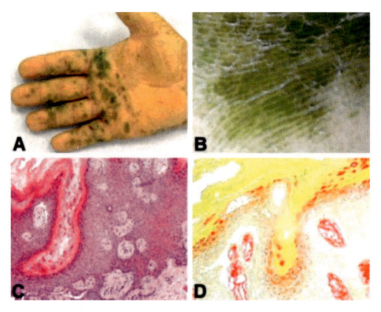

Bleeding Diathesis

This is one reason it is important not to let the blood be too viscous.

Chemistry Tests are commonly performed from blood serum, we add a specific chemical ("reagent") to the serum that reacts with the substance of interest-- and goes on to form a certain shade of color in the serum.

We analyze how deep this shade is with a **spectrophotometer**, and compare it to known shades for known amounts.

Then we can elucidate just how much substance (**"concentration"**) there was in the original serum. Like hematology tests, chemistry tests are much cheaper to "batch" onto a large **"auto-analyzer"**; it often costs as much for one test "stat" as for **20 tests** on a **"routine panel"**.

The number of chemistry tests given on various panels is different between laboratories, as is the name of the panels.

It is usually something like **"SMA-6"** or "Chem Panel 20" where the number shows how many tests are being done.

The simplest panel usually contains the **"electrolytes"**-- sodium, potassium, chloride and bicarbonate-- as well as glucose and perhaps **Creatinine** or **BUN**.

These will be described below. More elaborate panels often give protein and cholesterol subtype breakdowns, enzymes released from damaged heart, kidneys or liver and even **thyroid function results (TFR)**.

"Toxicology" tests tell drug levels in the blood or urine. In general, chemistry tests take less than 1 day and can be run "stat" within an hour:

Sodium is the salt of the blood. Water tends to follow this substance.

Electrolyte means something that **assists** electricity in traveling across a fluid, and sodium is our most plentiful electrolyte.

Normal sodium is between 135 - 148 milliequivalents per liter (meq/L) of blood.

When sodium is too **high** it is called "**hypernatremia**", this can be due to dehydration or excessive salt intake with poor kidney function. Low sodium, called "**hyponatremia**" is more commonly seen in cancer patients.

It can be due to the **SIADH** syndrome (Syndrome of Inappropriate secretion of anti-diuretic Hormone) which causes a lot of **water retention** in the blood with dilution of the sodium there.

SIADH is seen with expanding brain tumors and some Small Cell Lung Cancers.

Abnormal sodium can be corrected with intravenous fluids, if it goes severely out of normal range it will lead to stupor, coma and death.

When the blood is too viscous, (the less viscous something is, the greater its ease of movement **fluidity**).

Sodium will be **increased;** when it is to **dilute** then it will be **decreased**.

The patient with PV and **"hemoconcentration"** (too concentrated a blood cell mass in the circulating blood) may be intravenous fluids for dilution.

Potassium is the **salt** of the body cells; it is high within blood cells but low in the serum-- exactly opposite sodium's concentrations.

Like sodium, it is an electrolyte. **Potassium** must stay delicately **balanced in the blood**.

Normal potassium is 3.5 - 5.2 meq/L. **High potassium** is called **"hyperkalemia"** and occurs with kidney failure, lack of insulin production, bursting of blood cells, increasing acidity of the blood, and by taking too much supplemental potassium.

Normally excess potassium in the bloodstream is forced into the blood cells by insulin, along with glucose.

With kidney failure the blood becomes more acidic, and potassium leaks of the body cells.

One of the important features of dialysis is to correct hyperkalemia and too much acidity of the blood (**"acidemia"**).

Too **low potassium** is "hypokalemia" and is common in patients taking **heart medicines**, taking diuretics which leech out potassium **flowing through the kidneys**, and in malnourished patients.

If potassium is either too **high or low** it **interferes** with the contractions of the muscles, and most worrisome is abnormal heartbeats or even heart attacks from abnormal potassium.

Low potassium can be corrected by supplemental pills, we are careful not to give (**push**) them **too fast** (e.g. more than 80 MEQ/ day) to avoid overshooting.

High potassium can be lowered by fluids, "**Kayexalate**", **Lasix diuretic** and **insulin** (in the hospital!).

In PV, there are many more blood cells than normal, and these cells are **high in potassium** within them.

If they burst too quickly (such as when chemotherapy is given), then it may dangerously increase blood potassium, so this is monitored.

Chloride, from chlorine, is the **negative** "counter-ion" that electrically **balances** the positive **charges of sodium and potassium**; it is also an **electrolyte**.

Normal chloride is 98 - 108 meq/L, which adds up to less than the sodium and potassium.

The rest of the electrolyte balance is made up of **"Bicarbonate"** and a few other ions like phosphate and sulfate.

The difference between the sodium plus potassium and the chloride plus bicarbonate is called the **"anion gap"** and increases if there is too much acidity to the blood, such as from taking excess vitamin C or aspirin.

Too **high Chloride** is called **"hyperchloremia"** and too low is **"hypochloremia"**, these are most commonly found along with sodium and potassium abnormalities.

When chloride is too **low** it may be from excess bicarbonate and dehydration, called **"contraction alkalosis"**.

Implanting the draining ureters into the bowel after (after bladder cancer has forced removal of the bladder) disturbs blood chloride from excess absorption.

Abnormal chloride is commonly corrected along with potassium and sodium.

Bicarbonate is the other negative counter-ion to the positive potassium and sodium, as mentioned above.

It is crucial for keeping the acid-base balance of blood.

Normal bicarbonate is 22 to 30 meq/L and is crucial for **balancing** the **acidic carbonic acid** formed when carbon dioxide is dissolved in the blood water.

Recall that we breath oxygen and combust carbon molecules from the food we take in to generate carbon dioxide, which is then breathed out.

If excess acid accumulates in the body, it is called **"acidosis"**.

Excess base is called **"alkalosis"**. The cause of these can be either **"metabolic"** or **"respiratory"**.

Metabolic means **from the kidneys** (or another source); they produce bicarbonate to balance the acidic tendencies of the blood.

Respiratory means from breathing out **too much** or **too little** carbon dioxide. If we cannot breathe well, say from severe asthma or Chronic Obstructive Pulmonary Disease (**COPD**), then carbon dioxide builds up in the blood, turning it more acidic.

The **kidneys** try to **compensate** by manufacturing more bicarbonate to balance the acid.

Conversely, if we are rapidly breathing ("**hyperventilating**") then over time the blood becomes to **alkaline**; the kidneys will then produce **less bicarbonate** and dump existing bicarbonate into the urine to compensate.

It is common for patients with kidney failure on dialysis to require **extra bicarbonate ampules to balance** the excess acid in their blood.

Also, when patients stop breathing are we are attempting resuscitation, bicarbonate may be administered to counteract the progressive increase in blood acidity as soon as breathing has stopped.

Too much acid or alkali in the blood eventually results in other electrolyte imbalance (particularly potassium), stupor, coma and death.

Creatinine is a substance put out by the muscles of the body and filtered by the kidneys, it normally ranges between 0.2 and 1.3 milligrams per deciliter.

When increased, it can indicate kidney damage. In fact, for every doubling of **creatinine value**, there is a halving of kidney function.

In long term PV, the kidneys can be damaged by hemoglobin released from fractured RBC's, uric acid (see below) dehydration and other factors.

Creatinine is particularly important to compare with the BUN (below) to determine whether the patient is dehydrated or not.

BUN is Blood Urea Nitrogen, it is **made from conjugation of ammonias released by proteins digested in the liver**.

The importance of BUN is that it will **go up** if there are a lot of blood cells being **broken down**, and if the patient is dehydrated.

A **Normal BUN** is between 5 and 20 milligrams per deciliter of blood. In diagnosing PV, we want to rule out that the increased hemoglobin and hematocrit is simply due to chronic dehydration.

We look at the **BUN to Creatinine ratio**-- if it is more than 20, it indicates possible dehydration and "relative polycythemia".

Uric Acid is released from cells as they are broken down and normally excreted by the kidneys. If the uric acid builds up in tissues, it can crystallize **causing gout.**

Long term **excess uric acid** being processed by the kidneys can damage them, causing **"urate nephropathy"** and **kidney stones**.

PV patients are thus prone to gout and kidney stones.

Fortunately, medications to help the kidneys excrete uric acid (**"allopurinal"**) and to reduce the inflammation of gout (**"cholchicine"**) are readily available.

Other Tests:

Arterial Blood Gas ("ABG") -- This test is important to **determine how** well **oxygen** is being **absorbed by the lungs** into the **bloodstream**, and how effectively carbon dioxide is being expelled.

We can use this test to help **rule-out** (RO) or **confirm** PV, since **poor absorption** of oxygen from the lungs or poor blood pumping by a weak heart **will** also **raise** the RBCs.

Disturbances of blood gases, such as low oxygen or retained carbon dioxide result in fatigue and acid-base disturbances of blood.

The **"ABG"** test is typically done by inserting a syringe into the radial artery of the wrist, as opposed to the venous blood used for other blood tests.

Ideally, it should immediately be obvious that arterial blood has been drawn, since it is of **brighter red** color than deoxygenated venous blood.

It is extremely important to apply proper pressure to the artery afterwards to **stop bleeding**.

Failure to do so can **interrupt the blood supply** the extremity it was drawn from.

This is why we **discourage** arterial blood draws (though often it is easier to find a pulsating artery than a relatively flat vein) for tests **except** the **Arterial Blood Gas** (ABG).

Lung and Heart Function Tests-- As noted above, poor heart or lung function will **cause** a **reflex increase** in RBC's, to carry forth whatever oxygen is available.

If the diagnosis is in doubt, we perform a "**Pulmonary Function Tests**" (PFT) that will **describe** how **well oxygen is diffused** through the lung membrane.

Long term use of tobacco or industrial exposures to soot can reduce the "**diffusion capacity**" of the lungs, **raising** RBC production.

So too can **poor heart function** reduce ability of blood to get where it needs to be-- the tissues-- causing them to "**cry out**" for **more oxygen** and hormonally **raising RBC** production.

If necessary, a thallium stress test or (Multi Gated Acquisition Scan) "**MUGA** "can test the heart's efficiency ("**cardiac function**").

Kidney Imaging-- Rarely, a **kidney tumor** can **increase RBC** production, this is since the kidney produces the **erythropoietin hormone that** stimulates the marrow to crank out new RBC's.

A **CT scan** of the kidneys, and/or **Intravenous Pyelogram** that

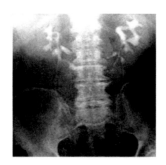
Intravenous Pyelogram

images them, will effectively rule-out whether a kidney tumor is the problem.

Erythropoietin Levels-- In heart, lung or kidney problems, the **increase** in RBC will be attributable to elevated erythropoietin hormone.

In PV, this hormone is typically **DECREASED**. This is due to the marrow sending a back a **Chromium -51** labeled Autologous RBC's-- If the cause of the **increased red blood cell** mass remains elusive, we can determine the **actual concentration** of

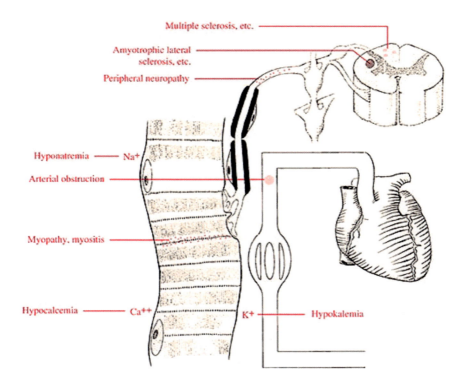

RBC's separate from dilutional or dehydration concerns. To do this, we extract out a known quantity of RBC's (simple blood draw), label them with a radioactive isotope as a marker, and then inject them back into the bloodstream.

We can then take a **new blood** sample, allowing time for the labeled RBC's to be distributed. By assessing the concentration of labeled RBC's in our new sample, we can calculate the **total RBC mass** in the body.

Hematocrits of over 60 are rarely just due to decreased plasma volume (plasma is the liquid portion of the blood).

For hematocrits of 50 - 60, where the diagnosis remains in doubt, this test can help.

Bone Marrow Biopsy -- This test is listed under **"hematology"** since we are looking at the blood forming elements of the bone.

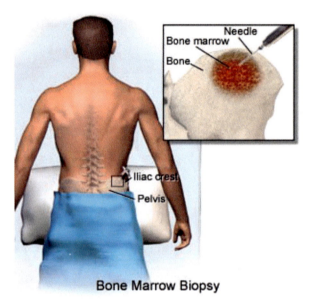

Bone Marrow Biopsy

The only way to diagnose many leukemias, and whether other cancers (like **Hodgkin's Disease** or **Small Cell Lung Cancer**) have spread to the bone marrow is by biopsy.

A **small core of bone and marrow** is taken with a **boring needle** from the hip wing(s) above the buttocks, see picture above, under local anesthetic.

The test can be uncomfortable but is **NOT** dangerous.

The **bone marrow removed** is suspended in preservative solution and smeared onto microscope slides for a **Differential**.

The bone marrow **looks different** than the circulating blood since the cells are less mature.

All blood cells originate from primordial **"Pleuripotential Stem Cells"** in the marrow, the process of **"differentiation"** turns them into various WBC's, RBC's and Platelets.

From an examination of the bone marrow, we can determine what the **circulating blood** will look like at later times, as the cells mature and are released.

We can also identify spread of other cancers into the marrow.

By doing a "**bilateral**" bone marrow biopsies (**both hips**) is about 15% **more accurate** than just doing one.

In PV, we expect to **see** a very **cellular** ("**hypercellular**") bone marrow, **cramped with new blood cells**, early in the disease.

Later, the overworked marrow tends to scar up (undergo **"fibrosis"**) and then fewer than normal cells are seen (**"hypocellular"**).

Sampled cells can be sent to look for characteristic chromosomal abnormalities.

What is the Natural Course of Polycythemia Vera?

Since the disease has a predilection to **patients older than 50** years old, it is most common for **patients** to **die** with, rather than from, the disease-- especially if it is properly treated.

It is usual for patients to have other medical problems (**"co-morbid conditions"**) like heart and lung disease to which they succumb first.

Most patients die of **"vascular complications"** (e.g. heart attack, stroke) of the disease, or of unrelated causes.

Over time, about 20% of patients **"progress"** to marked spleen enlargement, anemia, and scarring ("fibrosis") of the bone marrow.

This is called the **"spent phase"** of the disease. Some researchers believe that **ALL** patients will eventually enter the **"spent phase"**-- if they live long enough.

As mentioned, many patients only **have partial manifestations** of the disease, which can stretch out over many years.

However, once the diagnosis is made, it is crucial to consider treatment (discussed below).

If **no treatment** is give, the average **survival is only 2 years**.

With treatment survival is commonly extended to over 10 years. An important drawback of aggressive treatment is a rise in the later rates of acute leukemia.

Without chemotherapy or radiation therapy, the risk of leukemia with PV **is** just **1-2%**.

However, if these are given then the leukemia **risk jumps to 15 - 20%**.

These later leukemias are **very refractory** to treatment and **tend to be** quickly **lethal**.

As will be seen, newer aggressive treatments are less likely to markedly increase leukemia risk, while still extending overall survival times.

What was the Historical Treatment for Polycythemia Vera?

The historical, effective treatment for PV was **"phlebotomy"**-- that is **letting out** excessive **blood** through an arm vein.

The procedure is identical to donating blood for the Red Cross, and is extremely safe when done properly.

Interestingly, phlebotomy was a treatment for many illnesses used by **medieval** physicians-- they wanted to **let out** the pent up **"poisonous humors"** in the body.

It was generally **useless**, and **often harmful**, especially in anemic or dehydrated patients.

Leeches were a way of causing slow bloodletting, or a cut was made in a vein.

The treatment did often give apparent **benefit**s for patients with **congestive heart failure**, who have backup of blood into the limbs and lungs, and a similar "**plethoric**" appearance in the face as PV patients.

It might also temporarily benefit patients with very high blood pressure, reducing headache, heart attack and stroke risk.

The usefulness of bloodletting is now confined to PV, where the average **life span** has been **increased from 2 to 12** years with phlebotomy alone.

Phlebotomy is not a "**cure**" but rather a therapy for the disease.

Letting out the excess RBC's lowers the hematocrit and hemoglobin levels, causing improvement in plethora, headache, ear ringing ("**tinitus**"), fatigue, visual disturbances, dizziness, and other myriad manifestations of the disease.

It can also **reduce** the viscosity of the blood, and **lessen** the changes of spontaneous blood clots ("**thrombosis**") leading to heart attack or stroke.

The **lost blood volume** is replaced by drinking fluids, and this helps further **dilute the blood**.

There may be some reduction in spleen size with proper phlebotomy, but part of the reason that the spleen gets enlarged is that it may become an area of RBC production outside the bone marrow-- that is so called "**extramedullary hematopoeisis**".

There are actually **areas in the spleen** and **liver** which start forming **new RBC's**-- especially as the bone marrow becomes more fibrotic and **"burnt-out"**.

Thus the spleen remains **enlarged in 75**% of patients with the disease.

Phlebotomy has great benefits of improving signs and symptoms of the disease, **extending lifespan**, and **not raising** leukemia risk as is seen with other therapies.

The later leukemia risk with phlebotomy alone is 1-2%-- the **same** as in a patient receiving **no treatment**.

The frequency of phlebotomy will vary with the particular patient-- it is typically monthly to every six months.

It takes **only an hour** or so **in the physician's office**. The times to do phlebotomy can be determined by the CBC results and level of symptoms.

Phlebotomy **is** a **simple, safe, time-tested** and **effective treatment** for PV.

It proportionately **removes all** the excess cells being produced in PV-- RBC's, WBC's and platelets.

Other newer treatments discussed below must be compared to phlebotomy when considering their effectiveness, side-effects and overall safety.

Sometimes **phlebotomy is crucial**. Phlebotomy remains the "**gold standard**" with which to compare the usefulness of **newer treatments.**

The **therapeutic options** for PV have **increased** over the past three decades, but their net effect on improving **survival remains** debatable.

Part of the reason for this is that when we consider life expectancy with PV, we are also considering all other possible diseases that mostly elderly patients will succumb to.

When we say that the survival with phlebotomy alone is 10 - 12 years, it means we are also including death from heart attacks, kidney failure, car accidents etc. into that survival statistic.

While **thrombotic events** (e.g. heart attacks and strokes) may be increased secondary to PV, they may also have occurred in the absence of this disease.

That is, **standard survival statistics** include mortality from all causes, whether related to the disease in question or not.

Also, certain treatments may **INCREASE** the chance for early death by virtue of their side effects.

Thus we must very carefully consider the risks and benefits and newer treatments before recommending them to a specific patient.

The **basic treatment** strategies **for PV** involve **reducing** the excess RBC burden-- since that is the **main cause** of clinical problems.

The strategies involve **three ways** of doing this–
1) **Phlebotomy,**
2) **Chemotherapy**
3) **Radioactive nuclides**.

They may be **used alone or** in **combination**.

Phlebotomy was discussed in the previous section, and continues to be a widely used and effective treatment for the disease.

Chemotherapy involves using chemicals to suppress the bone marrow, so less of all blood cell types are produced.

Interestingly, this **"bone marrow suppression"** by chemotherapy is generally an **undesirable side effect** when using chemicals to treat cancer-- since it causes the classic side-effects of anemia, fatigue, easy bruising and increased infection risk.

However, in treating PV with chemotherapy, we are actually **utilizing** the **side-effects of chemotherapy** for a therapeutic purpose!

Nonetheless, chemotherapy **must be** strictly monitored to ensure that we do not "over-suppress" the marrow causing **severe side-effects ("toxicity")**.

Radiation therapy is also a potent suppressor of the bone marrow-- especially when the whole body is irradiation **TBI** ("Total Body Irradiation"). Instead of using classical **"External Beam"** irradiation, which gives **high doses** to the skin and organs, we use special radioactive chemicals, particularly **Phosphorus-32**.

This **"radionuclide"** is **injected** into the bloodstream, and preferentially **circulates** into the **marrow to suppress** its production of new blood cells.

Both chemotherapy and radiation therapy are described in further detail below.

Chemotherapy was first used in the 1940's; the first chemotherapy **"agents"** used were called **"alkylating agents"** and **derived from mustard gas**.

Back in **World War I**, the use of this poisonous gas was seen to destroy victims bone marrow.

Those **affected** would **first** develop fevers from lack of **White Blood Cells (WBS)**, Then bruising from depletion of platelets, and finally (if they lived long enough) anemia from lack of RBC production by the injured bone marrow.

It was soon **realized** that the **preferential action** on bone marrow of mustard gas derivatives could be exploited to help **destroy** cancers of White Blood Cell origin (e.g. Hodgkin's disease, leukemias, lymphomas).

The alkylating agents were popularized with the observation that they could sometimes cure White Blood Cell cancers, albeit they **did have serious** adverse **side effects**-- owing to their global suppression of the bone marrow.

They were **NOT** specific for cancer cells, but seemed to **kill** them at a **quicker rate** than normal cells.

This difference accounted for their clinical **usefulness**-- but they were dosed **very cautiously** ("**titrated**") to be **safe**.

Various Alkylating agents **were tried** for **treating PV**.

They Include:

1) Melphalan
2) Busulfan
3) Cyclophosphamide ("Cytoxan")
4) Cis
5) CarboPlatin
6) BCNU
7) CCNU
8) Dacarbazine
9) Procarbazine
10) Mechlorethamine

11) Ifosphamide.

They all "**alkylate**" the **DNA**, which **means add** a methyl or ethyl group, resulting in a "**chain termination**" when the DNA tries to divide-- that is a **useless** fragment of **DNA** instead of the whole necessary piece.

Since they are not specific for any particular cells, they have this effect on any quickly dividing cells in the body.

Alkylators produce "**bone marrow suppression**" with **lowered Red Blood Cells ("anemia")**, which is the goal in PV.

However, they also lower ("**leucopenia**") leading to easy infections and platelets **White Blood Cells ("thrombocytopenia"**) causing easy bruising or internal bleeding.

The **combination of all** of these is called "**pancytopenia**".

BCNU and **CCNU** are used **primarily** for **brain tumors** since they **penetrate** through the protective **blood-brain barrier.**

Cyclophosphamide and the similar **Ifosphamide** can **cause sloughing** of the bladder's inner lining (called **"hemorrhagic cystitis"**) which can be partly prevented by using the drug **MESA** which is a **"uroprotectant"**).

They also **cause** more **scalp baldness ("alopecia")** than the other alkylators.

Cisplatin (more than Carboplatin) **causes nerve damage**, first felt as numbness in the toes and progressing upward **("peripheral neuropathy")**, as well as decreased hearing.

It also **causes kidney** damage **("nephrotoxicity")**, the dose should be **reduced** if kidney or liver damage are present to avoid excess buildup of the drug in the bloodstream.

Busulphan can **cause** a syndrome resembling **lung scarring** and **malfunction** of the **adrenal glands**.

As a **"Late"** effect (if occurs it averages 10 years after treatment) some patients get **"non-lymphocytic leukemias"** which tend to be very aggressive.

They are somewhat more likely if patients get radiation also.

The **rate of** later **leukemias** in PV patients getting alkylating agents is as **high as 20%** in some studies.

The tendency of a drug to **cause** later leukemias means it's **"leukemogenic"**.

Some alklyators can be **taken by mouth** (e.g. Busulfan, CCNU, Cytoxan).

These are the ones most commonly used in PV treatment. For the ones that can't, leakage of the IV into the skin can cause local tissue damage.

Another type of **chemotherapy** agent used for PV are the **"antimetabolites"**, these were developed after the alkylating agents.

They are used more commonly **owing** to **less** propensity to be **"leukemogenic"**-- that is less chance of causing later leukemia.

These drugs have been supplanting the alkylating agents over the past 15 years.

Various **Anti-metabolites** have been **tried for treating** PV. These include: Hydroxyurea (hydrea-- very common), 6-Mercaptopurine, Methotrexate, Thiotepa Cytarabine

("ARA-C"), Cladribine, and 5-Fluorouracil (with/without leucovorin).

They **interfere with DNA** and protein synthesis by **"pretending"** to be something they are not, such as 1 of the 5 needed bases (RNA has Aerosol); this **"Trojan horse"** results in a **useless** product being synthesized, or a premature end to a product (**"chain termination"**).

They are called **"anti-metabolites"** since they **compete** with normal **metabolites**.

Again, it does this to any **quickly dividing cells**.

Anti-metabolites interfere with quickly dividing cells, so the patient will see pancytopenia, nausea and vomiting, mouth soreness, and peripheral nerve damage (from damage to "myelin", the insulating coating of the long nerve processes that keeps them from short-circuiting).

The affect on white blood cells (as with the other bone-marrow suppressing anti-neoplastic agents) can cause a marked decrease in the germ fighting **"neutrophil"** white cells, this is called **"neutropenia"**.

If a fever develops with this, it is called **"febrile neutropenia"** and this is a **medical emergency**; the patient requires **antibiotics immediately or** may **die**.

This is since the body's ability to fight infection is so low when **neutropenic** (less than 1000 neutrophils per milliliter of blood).

Usually, **three** complementary **intravenous antibiotics** are given for febrile neutropenia, and the patient will not be released from the hospital until the fever is manageable **("afebrile")**.

As with the alklylating agents, some anti-metabolites **can** be taken by mouth (e.g. methotrexate, hydroxyurea, 6-MP).

Hydroxyurea ("Hydrea") used in oral doses of 1 to 3 grams per day is currently the **drug of choice** for most patients in whom chemotherapy is utilized.

It does not appear to **increase** later **leukemia risk**. It helps **control** the symptoms of elevated metabolism, but has **more effect** on elevated WBC and platelet counts than on RBC's.

As such, **occasional phlebotomy** is commonly required in addition to this chemotherapy.

As mentioned above, it must be **carefully titrated** and monitored so that **immune function** is not too severely depressed by the depletion of WBC's.

This will require periodic **Complete Blood Counts** ("CBC") to check the blood cell status.

Using Hydroxyurea may **increase survival** compared to phlebotomy alone, as noted in the European Cooperative Group Studies.

The indications for using chemotherapy are discussed more fully in the Comparison of Therapies section ahead.

Radiation Therapy has been used since 1940, with injected forms of radioactive isotopes being the preferred method of administration.

It was found that the radionuclide **Phosphorus-32** preferentially **gravitated to bone marrow** (the bones have a propensity to absorb phosphorus and calcium).

The administration of **Phosphorus-32** is easy; it is simply injected into an arm vein in the Nuclear Medicine Department of a hospital.

It provides long, trouble free **remissions from PV** in most cases, and **successfully reduces** signs and symptoms of the disease.

The dose given is commonly 85.2 MBq ("MegaBequerals") of Phosphorus-32 per **"square meter"** of patient body surface area.

Most people have between 1.2 - 2.0 square meters of skin surface area. The patient is then closely followed with **Complete Blood Counts** for 3 months, and retreated (if needed) with a dose 25% greater than the initial dose.

This can be further **repeated** after 3 more months, but is **rarely necessary**.

The typical remission with Phosphorus-32 **lasts between 1 and 2 years,** during which the patient is commonly **symptom-free**.

The **Phosphorus-32** therapy may be repeated if relapse occurs.

One serious concern is the **increased risk** for developing leukemia when Phosphorus-32 is used; this risk is as **high as** 15% in some studies.

While this means that 85% of patients **avoid this problem**, those who **get leukemia will** almost inevitably **die** from it.

Higher total dose of Phosphorus-32, repeat treatments, and simultaneous chemotherapy increase risk.

As with chemotherapy discussed above, suppression of bone marrow function with Phosphorus-32 can have undesired side effects. If the degree of suppression is too great, then the patient can develop intractable anemia, consistently low WBC counts causing immune system malfunction, and low platelet counts with resultant easy bruising and internal bleeding risk.

Thus the dose of **Phosphorus-32** must be carefully titrated with an **eye on blood counts** to avoid "**overshooting**" and annihilating the necessary bone marrow.

There may be a **"delayed recovery"** of months to years after radioisotope administration, or sufficient recovery may never occur.

If the bone marrow is irreversibly **damaged**, it leads to **"pancytopenia"** meaning that all crucial blood cells will be low.

Bone marrow **"aplasia"** means that the marrow is **destroyed.** If this occurs, then the patient **will need** regular **transfusions** or a bone marrow transplant procedure to live.

However, it is extremely unlikely from therapeutic doses of chemotherapy or Phosphorus-32.

The more common cause of bone marrow aplasia over time in PV is a **"burnt out"**, fibrotic marrow that has been replaced by scar tissue.

In this situation of **advanced PV**, paradoxically RBC and platelet transfusions may be needed to sustain life-- since the marrow **has** finally **failed.**

Phosphorus-32 puts out a gamma ray with a maximum energy of **1.7 Megavolts**, this is somewhat **more penetrating than Cobalt-60** (which is 1.25 Megavolts).

The **radiation** emitted **falls off** very **quickly** from where the Phosphorus-32 is located, and so it is negligible at a foot or so away from the patient.

The time is takes for half of the isotope to **"decay"** (lose radioactivity) is called **"half-life"**; for phosphorus-32 it is

14.3 days.

Thus, **99%** of the isotope **is gone** after 10 half lives (143 days).

The isotope is rapidly absorbed into bone; some is also excreted into the urine.

You can see that it is relatively long lasting in the bone.

It is advisable, for **extra caution**, for patients who get **Nuclear Isotopes** to **avoid** holding small **children** for several weeks.

The very young are more **susceptible** to later cancers from low dose radiation exposure than adults.

In general though, Phosphorus-32 is a safe and effective therapy for getting most patients with PV into remission. It is only the tendency for increasing leukemias that prevents its more frequent use.

Comparison of Therapies:

Studies comparing treatments for PV have been performed by the **Polycythemia Vera Study Group** and the results published through the past two decades.

In a landmark study, this group randomly assigned patients to one of three therapies:

1) Phlebotomy Alone-- This was discussed above and represents **safe and effective therapy** for PV.

As is seen from the other "**arms**" of the Polycythmia Vera Study Group below, it is **often necessary** to use **Phlebotomy** in conjunction with **Chemotherapy** and **Radiation Therapy--** since those treatments may not sufficiently reduce Red Blood Cell mass quickly enough.

If a **PV** patient goes for **emergency surgery** (**coronary angioplasty** is common example) then it is **CRUCIAL** that they be properly phlebotomized (bled) to control Red Blood Cell mass prior to surgery.

If Red Blood Cell mass is **NOT** properly controlled prior to surgery, then the **death rate** from surgery is 4 - 5 times higher than in patients properly controlled (phlebotomized) prior to surgery.

Fluid **"plasma expanders"** can be put in to avoid too rapid a diminution of blood volume that occurs with **rapid bleeding,** thus avoiding **low blood pressure** problems ("**hemodynamic instability**").

The most likely **side-effects** of **rapid Phlebotomy** are dizziness and nausea, much the same as when blood is donated for transfusions.

Side effects can be lessened by slower Phlebotomy, giving fluids, and possibly anti-nauseant (e.g. Compazine) or tranquilizer (e.g. Valium) pills prior to the procedure.

It is important the patients have had a **good breakfast** before going in for Phlebotomy, but eating a lot right before the procedure **isn't recommended** to reduce possible nausea.

Again, it is an **easy and safe** therapy to get which requires only about an hour in the clinic.

As mentioned above, **neither chemotherapy** nor **radiation therapy** are guaranteed to produce sufficient **decrease** in Red Blood Cell Mass-- and so at least occasional Phlebotomy is likely to be necessary anyway.

Phlebotomy remains the mainstay of both historic and current therapy for PV.

In the original Polycythemia Study Group trials, patients getting Phlebotomy alone were more likely to have **heart attacks or strokes** during the first four years of therapy, but after the seventh year the survival was **BETTER** with Phlebotomy alone, mostly due to leukemias from other therapy.

2) Chemotherapy and Phlebotomy-- Chemotherapy which depresses bone marrow function was tried in the International Polycythemia Group Studies, it was chosen to reflect what was being used in Oncologist's offices.

It was necessary, as discussed above, to supplement Chemotherapy with Phlebotomy to ensure that the Red Blood Cell mass was properly reduced. Chemotherapy is fickle, it has differering effects in different patients.

Some patients **tolerate Chemotherapy** very well, and have **little** or **no side effects**, and an **excellent overall result**.

However, other patients are inexplicably **stricken** with all sorts of side effects, tolerate the treatment poorly, and/or don't get satisfactory results.

Treatment must therefore be **individualized**; the chemotherapy agent chosen is very **carefully adjusted** ("") to give optimal effects.

In the original Polycythemia **titrated"** Group Studies, the agents **used** were **either Melphalan**, **Busulfan**, or **Chlorambucil**-- they were all Alkylating agents.

Chlorambucil was **dropped** since over 10% of patients being treated with it later developed leukemia-- it is **no longer recommended.**

Busulfan remains somewhat popular, although it can cause a syndrome resembling lung scarring ("**pulmonary fibrosis**") with difficulty breathing.

The **syndrome** commonly **improves**, but does **not** totally resolve, when **Busulfan** is discontinued.

The dose for **Busulfan** is usually 4 to 6 milligrams per day by mouth; however the **effect is more** on lowering platelets and White Blood Cells than RBC's.

Thus **Phlebotomy** is also added as needed. Again, there is a later leukemia **risk** from Busulfan or any Alkylating Agent.

The **best** current **Chemotherapy agent is Hydroxyurea**, this "**Hydrea**" is also **given by mouth** and is **not known** to **cause leukemia**.

It is given in doses of 1 - 3 milligrams per day by mouth titrated by blood counts.

In the original Polycythemia Study Group Trials, patients who got Chemotherapy had overall **POORER survival** than those who didn't.

Part of this was due to some patients **having more** aggressive PV disease and so requiring more treatment.

However, European studies have shown **IMPROVED** survival and normal leukemia risk in those patients getting new Chemotherapy, compared to Phlebotomy alone.

3) Phosphorus-32 and Phlebotomy-- As mentioned, marrow suppression with **Phosphorus-32** isotope is **easy**, provides **long** and **problem-free remissions** in most cases, and **reduces** the signs and **symptoms of PV**.

It may be **repeated** as necessary, stimulating a new remission.

The duration of successive remissions **does tend** to be **shorter** than the initial remission.

In a Polycythemia Study Group Trials, 85.2 MegaBequerals (MBq) of the isotope per square meter of patient's body surface area were injected into a vein in the Nuclear Medicine Department.

The **effect of** the **Phosphorus-32** was **not** immediate, but took weeks to a couple of months to plateau.

During this time, and periodically thereafter, patients **still required Phlebotomy for reductive** of excessive Red Blood Cell mass.

The worst complication of Phosphorus-32 is a higher risk for later leukemias, refractory to cure.

An analysis of a large number of patients getting Phosphorus-32 showed leukemia risk of about 15%, while **NOT ENHANCING SURVIVAL OVER OTHER FORMS OF THERAPY.**

Again, the risk of leukemia is related to the total dose of Phosphorus-32 given over time, so it is increased with repeated treatments.

Also, the longer patients **live after treatment**, the **more** chance they have to develop leukemia.

Thus, Phosphorus-32 should **only be** considered **for elderly patients** who do not have a very long (>5 years) life expectancy owing to other medical conditions.

In these patients Phosphorus-32 can be relatively safe, effective therapy that reduces symptoms and the need for frequent Phlebotomy.

Some More Things To Consider:

Since most early deaths from the disease are due to clotting events (like heart attack or stroke) it may be **advisable** to take a mild dose of aspirin (such as an 80 mg. children's aspirin) daily to help **"thin the blood"**.

Large studies have shown that this **reduces clotting** ("**thrombotic**") events in the general population, and it should be especially helpful for PV patients.

It is **important** to **avoid** becoming **dehydrated**, as this further **increases** the viscosity of the blood and the risk for clots.

Drinking about 6 glasses of water per day (presuming normal kidney and heart function) helps keep the blood "**thinner**" and preserve normal kidney function by flushing out contaminants.

It is also **important to change diet** to reduce cholesterol if it is elevated, and get enough vitamins and minerals.

It is further **crucial** to get a reasonable amount of exercise to assist circulation and relieve stress.

These habits will reduce complications from PV, **reduce** odds for other medical problems, and enhance the general quality of life.

The following Members have been certified by the **Association for Meridian Energy Therapies** (The AMT) as Meridian Energy Therapy Practitioners. This qualification also includes intensive knowledge of Emotional Freedom Techniques (EFT).

Zeinab Abdel — Advanced Practitioner — Cairo, Egypt

Sahar Fouad Abdel Hay — Advanced Practitioner — Cairo, Egypt

Noel Abel — Staffordshire, United Kingdom

Maude Allen — Minnesota, United States

Sonia Amills — Advanced Practitioner — Wiltshire, England

Shirley Andreas — Buckinghamshire, United Kingdom

Danica Apolline   Middlesex, England

Mark Atkinson   Advanced Practitioner London, England

Jennie Baker   Lancashire, England

Julie Ball   Kent, England

Varda Banilivy   Trainer New York, United States

Sassona Baron   British Columbia, Canada

Jayne Bartlett   Advanced Practitioner Hampshire, England

Paula Bennett   Leicestershire,
        England

Irene Bennett
        England

Kiren Bhogal   West Midlands,
        England

Sarah Bird   County Wicklow,
        Ireland

Carol Borthwick   Provence,
        France

Caroline Bottrill   Derbyshire,
        United Kingdom

Kim Bradley   London,
        England

Ruth Bray   Co Cork,
        Ireland

Alan Bridges   Asturias,
        Spain

Claire Brown   Somerset,
        United Kingdom

Doug Buckingham   London,
        England

Alan Burbanks   East Yorkshire,
        United Kingdom

Nigel Burgan   Surrey,
        England

Pauline Campbell   Glasgow,
        Scotland

Sally Canning   Nottinghamshire,

          England

Malcolm Caple   West Midlands,

          United Kingdom

John Castle   Essex,

          England

Serena Chancellor   Northamptonshire,

          England

Margaret Chenoweth   South Wales,

          Wales

Keith Cherrington   South Gloucestershire,

          England

Julie Cheshire

          England

Mary Chesters — Leicestershire, England

Elizabeth Child — West Midlands, England

Maggie Childs — Gloucestershire, United Kingdom

Sheila Cook — England

Helen Cook — Glasgow, Scotland

Barry Cooper — London, England

Lesley Court — Dubai, United Arab Emirates

Susan Courtney — Hampshire, England

Lesley Cox — East Yorkshire, United Kingdom

Sara Cureton — Shropshire, United Kingdom

Andrea Darcy Fretwell — Warwickshire, United Kingdom

Karl Dawson — Warwickshire, England

Ruth Dean — Warwickshire, United Kingdom

Janet Deane — Donegal, Ireland

Scott Degville — West Midlands, England

Peter Delves — Warwickshire, England

Monika Denes — Amstelveen, The Netherlands

Katie Dennington — Surrey, United Kingdom

Tony Dickinson — London, England

Sandra Dickson — Middlesex, England

Catherine Dixon — London, England

Helen Dolley — Warwickshire, England

Therese Doran — California, United States

David Dove — Oxon, England

Eilean Drysdale — Jaen, Spain

Jenny Dunn — Nottinghamshire, England

Sonja Eckl-Riel — Isle of Skye, Scotland

Nahla El Henawy — Cairo, Egypt

Amanda Elithorn — Surrey, England

Kate Elliott — County Down, Northern Ireland

Frances Emmett — Oxon, United Kingdom

June Eyre — Nottinghamshire, England

Marian Farrell — Co. Dublin, Ireland

Lorna Firth — Paphos, Cyprus

Therese Fitzgerald — County Down, Northern Ireland

Margarita Foley

    Ireland

Kjell Forsberg   Ystad (Peppinge),

    Sweden

Ann-Sofi Forsberg   Ystad (Peppinge),

    Sweden

Morag Foster M.A. PGDE   Advanced Practitioner

    England

Jolie-Ann Francis   North Somerset,

    United Kingdom

Deborah Gair   Hertfordshire,

    England

Kay Gire   Lancashire,

    England

Patricia Glasspool　　　　Hampshire, England

Debra Goldston　　　　Shropshire, England

Matthew Gray　　South Glamorgan,　　　　Wales

Donna Green　　　　Surrey, England

Markus Greus　　　　　　Boras, Sweden

Linda Gyllensvan　　　Varberg, Sweden

Janet Haddon　　　West Midlands, England

Maggie Hall — Derbyshire, England

Lynne Hancher — West Midlands, England

Barbara Handley — West Midlands, England

Jeanine Hanneman — Hampshire, England

Chrissie Hardisty — Cheshire, England

Carl Harrison — Bedfordshire, England

Gill Hartley — Surrey, England

Stella Haylett — Buckinghamshire, United Kingdom

Elizabeth Haylett Clark — London, United Kingdom

Birgitta Heiller — Surrey, England

Alison Hill — Worcestershire, England

Sandra Hillawi — Hampshire, England

Manisha Hirani — Middlesex, United Kingdom

Jane Hodgkin — London, United Kingdom

Paula Hogg   Edinburgh, Scotland

Elizabeth Hogon   London, England

Rosemary Homer   Bristol, England

Teri Howlett   Berkshire, England

Trudie Hudson   England

Heather Hull   Derbyshire, England

Valerie Ieronimo   Nottinghamshire, England

Kim Ingleby   Avon,

        England

Valerie Ives   West Midlands,

        England

Ulla Jacobsson   Hälsingland,

        Sweden

Denise Jacques

        England

Lynda Jakiro

        England

Svetlina Jeanneret   Cambridgeshire,

        England

Sara Jeffery   Kent,

        England

Clive Jelley — Derbyshire, United Kingdom

Heather Johnston — Co Antrim, Northern Ireland

Mary Jones — Buckinghamshire, England

Frances Jones — Avon, England

David Jones — England

Barbara Jones — Stockport, England

Mats Jonsson — Stockholm, Sweden

Gisela Kahler — Hampshire, England

Nirmla Mindy Kaur — West Midlands, United Kingdom

Nancy Kennewell — Nottinghamshire, England

Aisling Killoran — Dublin, Ireland

Sarah King — Warwickshire, United Kingdom

Cuneyt Konuralp — Istanbul, Turkey

Christiana Kriechbaum-Hinteregger — Croatia

Michael Kulyk   Middlesex,

            England

Irene Lambert   Derbyshire,

            England

Anthony Lambert

            England

Kirsten Larsen   Surrey,

            England

Clive Lawrence   Derbyshire,

            England

Peter Lee   Stokholm,

            Sweden

Mary Lissett   West Midlands,

            United Kingdom

Kimberley Lovell — Somerset, England

Cilla Lye — Stockholm, Sweden

Lauren Ann Maclennan — Wicklow, Ireland

Suzanne Manning — Berwickshire, Scotland

Ray Manning — Dublin, Ireland

John Marsh — Cheshire, England

Susan Martin — Northamptonshire, England

Elizabeth Mason Wiltshire,
England

Anne Mathews Steyning,
United Kingdom

Doris Mc Cann
Ireland

Sheona Mc Ewan Aerdenhout,
Netherlands

Dee McCall
England

Helen McCrarren Co Monaghan,
Ireland

Linda McCroft Norfolk,
England

Gillian McDonagh — Kent, United Kingdom

Suzanne McKeon — Dublin, Ireland

Donna McManus — Hertfordshire, United Kingdom

Jan Meldrum — Tyne And Wear, England

Alison Menzies — Eindhoven, Netherlands

Hayley Miller — Derbyshire, England

Michael Millett — London, England

Julie Milward   Derbyshire,
         England

Nicky Minter   Wiltshire,
         England

Phil Mollon   Hertfordshire,
         England

Dorothy Morris   Dublin,
         Ireland

Martha Morrison   County Louth,
         Ireland

Frances Moss   Essex,
         United Kingdom

Deirdre Mullen
         Ireland

Anne Mundkur	West Midlands, England

Dee Nanua	Derbyshire, United Kingdom

Pamela Neill	Isle Of Man, United Kingdom

Kathrine Nielsen	London, England

Trevor Noble	Hampshire, England

Mary O'Brien	Dublin, Ireland

Sarah O'Donnell	England

Sofia Olsson　　　　　　Stokholm,

　　　Sweden

James Orr　　　　　　　London,

　　　England

Bridie Page　　　　　　 Derbyshire,

　　　United Kingdom

Charlotte Palmgren　　　 Järfälla,

　　　Sweden

Elaine Parke　　　　　　Cardiff,

　　　Wales

Lorraine Parker　　　　　Derbyshire,

　　　United Kingdom

Sally Anne Parmar　　　 Derbyshire,

　　　United Kingdom

Charlotte Parr — East Yorkshire, United Kingdom

Andrew Alexander Parsons — Hertfordshire, United Kingdom

Frederick Passmore — Derbyshire, United Kingdom

Shilpa Patel — Middlesex, England

Nicola Phoenix — London, England

Lois Pimentel — London, England

Louise Player — North Somerset, England

Lilian Poultney   Leicestershire,

            England

Louise Prevost   Berkshire,

            England

Mel Prynne   Surrey,

            United Kingdom

Nicola Quinn   East Sussex,

            England

Timothy Quinn   East Sussex,

            England

Frank Quinton   Hampshire,

            England

Sandi Radomski   Pennsylvania,

            United States

Penny Rattle   Surrey,

    England

Robert Rawson   Derbyshire,

    United Kingdom

Andrew Reay   Victoria,

    Australia

Karen Rhodes   West Yorkshire,

    England

Judy Richardson   Cumbria,

    England

Hazel Riggall   West Midlands,

    United Kingdom

Gill Riley

    England

Rowana Rowan   Kent,
                      England

David Rowbotham   Edinburgh,
                      Scotland

Avril Rushton   Hampshire,
                      England

Helen Ryle   Co Kerry,
                      Ireland

Joy Salem   Hertfordshire,
                      England

Hilary Salt   Conwy,
                      Wales

Carole Samuda   Hants,
                      United Kingdom

Barbara Saph — Hampshire, England

Sereena Saroi — England

Jane Saunders — Hertfordshire, England

Nicola Saunders — Northamptonshire, England

Sue Sawyer — Hampshire, England

Heather Scothern — Nottinghamshire, England

Janice Scott — London, England

Stella Scott-Svedberg   Malmö, Sweden

Roma Shorthouse   Northmaptonshire, United Kingdom

Christine Sillett   Leicestershire, United Kingdom

Cathy Simmons   England

Maggie Skinner   West Midlands, England

Jim Small   Staffordshire, England

Rosemary Smith   Dorset, England

Lucia Solaz-Frasquet

England

Michael Somers — County Kildare,

Ireland

Gordon Soutar — Midlothian,

Scotland

Darren Stamford — London,

United Kingdom

Mary Stammers — Dublin 24,

Ireland

Anne Stanton — Yorkshire,

England

Janette Stoppard

England

Jane Stredder   Hampshire, England

Eileen Strong   Staffordshire, England

Steve Sullivan   Essex, England

Kenneth Svensson   Sverige, Sweden

Angela Swann   Gloucestershire, England

Anne Sweet   England

Beverli Taylor   Nottinghamshire, England

Duncan Tennant   West Lothian,

    Scotland

Lynne Theophanides   Cardiff,

    Wales

Parameswari Thiyagarajah   Shropshire,

    England

Kerry Thornback

    England

Stephena Thorne   Hampshire,

    England

Janice Tidy   Middlesex,

    England

Karen Tinker   Yorkshire,

    England

Peter Tomlinson   Lancashire,

           England

Stephen Tonry   Worcestershire,

           England

Deirdre Toohey   Co Galway,

           Ireland

Sally Topham   London,

           England

Jane Towse   East Yorkshire,

           United Kingdom

Robin Trewartha

           England

Barbara Trotter   Nelson,

           New Zealand

Mary Van Der Stam — Geldrop, Netherlands

Carol Vivyan — Channel Islands, United Kingdom

Allison Walker — England

Judith Walker — England

Emily Walsh — Dublin, Ireland

Joyce Waring — South Yorkshire, England

Maureen Warner — Derbyshire, United Kingdom

Shirley Warrington — Gloucestershire, England

Louise Waters — Hampshire, England

Kerin Webb — Dorset, England

Shirley Webb — Hertfordshire, England

Julie Wells — Suffolk, United Kingdom

Angela Western — Kent, England

Susan White — London, England

Tony Whitehead   Somerset,
                        England

Julia Wilson   Lancashire,
                        England

Patricia Wilson   Cornwall,
                        England

Rob Wood
                        England

Forbes Woodland   Warwickshire,
                        England

Julie Woods-Byrne   Dublin 3,
                        Ireland

Tom Wynn   Dublin,
                        Ireland

Reto Wyss   Berne, Switzerland

Barbara Zell

England

Poly MVA is a new, nontoxic, powerful antioxidant formula that **protects** both cellular DNA and RNA.

The scientifically designed mechanism of action is to "fix the cell" and control the cancer, rather than "fight the cancer" and poison the system as noted above.

Poly MVA offers an extremely powerful alternative cancer treatment without the toxic side effects associated with most Conventional Cancer Treatments.

Doctors (See Practioners List below) and **Patients worldwide** are reporting the benefits of **Poly MVA** when used as a stand-alone option or when used in conjunction with Chemotherapy and Radiation.

POLY MVA has been scientifically designed to **CORRECT DNA BREAKDOWNS** and return the damaged cell to normal cellular function.

This product was developed by **Dr. Merrill Garnett**, a highly regarded biochemist, who has been conducting research with the objective of creating an electronic frequency specificity to restore the DNA exchange energy pathway.

Poly-MVA(LAPd) compounds transfer current inward from the cell membrane phospholipid to DNA via the mitochondria.

This high flux state of inward pulsed current maintains normal electron oxygen transport, but can be shown to electrically dissociate (breakdown) membranes of primitive anaerobic (CANCER) cells including amoeba, yeasts, and certain tumors.

ALABAMA

Larry D. Brock, MD
Regenerative Medicine Center
5901 Airport Blvd. Suite E Mobile, Alabama 36608-3156
Ph:251-342-0505
Fax: 251-342-0360
email: drbrock@regenerativemedicine-al.com

Website: www.bioidenticalhormonemd.com

ALASKA

Gary Geraly, M.D.

615 East 82nd Ave., Suite 300

Anchorage, Alaska, 99518

Phone: (907)-344-7775

Fax: (907)-522-3114

E-Mail: compmed@alaska.net

ARIZONA

Lloyd Armold DO
Preventive & Family Medicine

7200 West Bell Rd

Suite G-103

Glendale, AZ 85308

Phone: 623-939-8916

Fax: (623) 486-8973

E-mail: doc@docarmold.com

John Black, D.C., Ph.D

1202 Willow Creek Road

Prescott, Arizona 86301

928-775-9508

E-Mail: drblack@highstream.net

Bryan T. McConnell, N.D.

170 N. La Canada #90

Green Valley, Arizona 85614

(520) 399-9212

Toll Free (877) 399-9212

E-Mail: thefirst_resort@msn.com

Stanley R. Olsztyn, M.D.

8580 E. Shea Blvd #110

Scottsdale AZ 85260

Phone: (480) 949-0500

E-Mail: srolsztyn@aol.com

Marnie Vail, M.D.

702 North Beaver Street

Flagstaff, Az. 86001

Phone: 928-214-9774

Fax: 928-214-9772

E-Mail: marnie@safeaccess.com

David C. Korn, D.O., D.D.S., M.D.(H)
LongLife Medical Incorporated

11518 East Apache Trail, Suite 115

Apache Junction, Az. 85220

Phone: 480-354-6700

E-Mail: information@long-life-medical.com

Website: www.long-life-medical.com

Robert Myers, N.D.

1000 Willow Creek, Suite E

Prescott, Arizona 86301

Phone: 928-445-1999

E-Mail: pinon@northlink.com

Jonathan Psenka ND
Christian Issels ND
Issels Medical Center

13832 N 32nd St. Suite 126

Phoenix, Arizona 85032

602-493-2273

E-mail: info@isselsmedicalcenter.com

Website: www.isselsmedicalcenter.com

Envita Natural Medical Centers of America

4614 E. Shea Blvd. Suite D #160

Phoenix, AZ 85028

Phone: 602-569-4144

Toll Free 1-866-830-4576

E-mail: staff@behealthyamerica.com

Website: http://behealthyamerica.com

Warren M. Levin, M.D., FAAFP, FACN, FAAEM
Issels Medical Center

13832 N. 32nd St. Suite 126
Phoenix, AZ 85032
Phone: 480-209-1846
Web Site: www.warrenmlevinmd.org

Thomas S. Lee, NMD, APH
NaturoDoc LLC, an online source of natural health products and consultations
1711 Stockton Hill Road #304
Kingman, AZ 86401

Phone: 928-767-4743 worldwide
Toll-free: 877-867-4743 from U.S. & Canada
Fax: 928-767-4643
Email: info@naturodoc.com
Website: www.naturodoc.com

Frank Sweet NMD
1731 Mesquite Ave Ste. 5
Lake Havasu City, AZ 86403
Phone: (928) 453-9525
Email: fpsweet@ctaz.com

Shivinder Deol , MD
Anti-Aging & Wellness Center
4000 Stockdale Hwy., Suite D
Bakersfield, CA 93309
Phone: (661) 325-7452
Fax: (661) 325-7456

E-mail: doc@drdeol.com

Website: http://www.drdeol.com

Areas of specialty: Alternative and complementary medicine. Diplomate, Anti-Aging Medicine. We use IV vitamin C, hyberbaric oxygen, pH balance, Poly-MVA and more to help support cancer patients.

Lauren Swerdloff MD
1821 Wilshire Blvd, Suite 220
Santa Monica, CA 90403
Office Phone: 310-829-5189
Office Fax: 310-829-5942

(Board Certified in Anti-Aging, Nutrient & Family Medicine, Specializing in Alternaive Medicine, Hormones, Nutrition and Thermography

---

ARKANSAS

CALIFORNIA

Andrea Cole-Raub, D.O.
Board Certified Family Practice

Board Certified Anti-Aging Medicine

Two Office Locations:

4510 Executive Drive

San Diego, Ca. 92121

858-535-1312

E-Mail: coleraub@cs.com

120 CravenRoad, Suite 207

San Marcos, Ca. 92078

760-510-8248

Kanti Makwana, N.D.

1611 Cabrillo Avenue

Torrance, Ca. 90501.

310 320 0319

E-mail: nutrimor@mediaone.net

Douglas K. Husbands, DC, CCN, ABAAHP

Athens Chiropractic Clinic

951 Industrial Road, Suite B

San Carlos, CA 94070

Phone: (650) 593-4447

Fax: (650) 593-5071

E-mail: inquiry@drhusbands.com

Website: www.drhusbands.com

Areas of specialty: Functional Health Care, Nutritional, and Anti-Aging Health Services. We offer comprehensive non-toxic therapies and modalities for a wide variety of integrative holistic health services. Advanced laboratory testing used for determining the underlying causes of disease and progression towards improvement. In-house Massage Therapy and Acupuncture services available.

Allan Sosin, M.D.
Institute for Progressive Medicine
16100 Sand Canyon Avenue, Suite 240
Irvine, Ca. 92618
Email: asosinmd@earthlink.net
Phone: 949-753-8889

Marc Weill,
CNC
Core Care Center
3023 Fillmore Street
San Francisco, Ca. 94123
Phone: 415-928-5423
E-Mail: cindy@corecarecenter.com
Website: http://www.corecarecenter.com

Robert Bolander MD We
Laurie Gentry, Coordinator
Mailing Address Only:
5149 Bluebell Ave.
North Hollywood, Ca. 91607
Phone: 310-455-0588
E-mail: mysticwave@knology.net

Maxine Wright PhD

9205 Redtail Hawk Lane
Cotati, California 94931
(Holistic, Metabolic Nutritionist
Located in the Santa Rosa, CA area)
Phone: 707-795-8791
E-mail: maxine@karunahealth.com

Effie Mae Buckley RN MN
Choice Healing
7174 Santa Teresa Blvd
Suite A6
San Jose, CA 95139
Phone: 408-363-1498
Email: choicehealing@aol.com

William S. Eidelman MD
The Center For Healing & Transformation
(Programs for Healing Serious Illnesses)
1654 N. Cahuenga Blvd.
Los Angeles, CA 90028
Phone: 323-463-3295
Fax: 323-463-3740
Email: williameidelman@gmail.com
Website: www.DrEidelman.com

Virginia Hernly DC
Chiropractic, Naturopathy, Nutrition
205 E 3rd Ave #406
San Mateo, CA 94401

Phone: 650 347 4443

Fax: 650 347 5783

Email: dr.vlhernly@sbcglobal.net

WebSite: www.creative-health.net

Alan Schwartz, MD
Holistic Resource Center
29020 Agoura Rd. #A8

Agoura Hills, CA 91301

Phone: (818) 597-0966

Donna South, ND

1143 Pinecrest Ave.

Escondido, CA 92025

Phone: (760) 839-0451

Fax: (760 747-5148

E-Mail: drdonnand250@cox.net

Dr. Robert Rowen
Dr. Terri Su
2220 County Center Dr. Suite H

Santa Rosa, CA 95403

707-545-5814

Dan Rogers MD, NMD
GersonPlus Therapy 710 E. San Ysidro Blvd. #485

San Ysidro, CA 92173

Phone: 646-435-2818

Email: DrRogers1@gmail.com

Website: www.gersonplus.com/

Comments:

I have been practicing Alternative Medicine for more than 30 years here in Tijuana, MX. I have also published in US Scientific Peer Reviewed Journals, and I am well known in the industry. I am also well known at NIH. I have been using Poly MVA for many years with my CA patients

Joshua Samanta, DC, CCSP, CSCS
Uptown Wellness Center
7354 Painter Ave.
Whittier, CA 90602
Phone: (562) 789-1999
Toll free: 866-935-8678
E-mail: UptownWellness@yahoo.com
Website: www.UptownWellness.com

COLORADO

Melanie Dailey, M.D.
James Dailey, N.D.
Rocky Mtn. Integrative Health
625 S. Lincoln Ave., Suite 206C
Steamboat Springs, Colorado 80487
Phone: 970-879-8569

E-Mail: melwind1@aol.com

Website: http://www.RMIHA.com

Annelle Norman, BSc (Hons) LCH

Vital Energy Clinic

3157 So. Broadway

Englewood, Colorado 80110

303-806-9114

720-854-1447 (cell and fax)

Terry Grossman, M.D., M.D.(H), N.M.D

Medical Director, Frontier Medical Institute

2801 Youngfield St, Ste. 117

Denver, Colorado 80401

Phone: 303-233-4247

Toll Free: 877-548-4387

Fax: 303-233-4249

E-Mail: customerservice@liv4evr.com

Website: http://www.liv4evr.com

Jonathan W. Singer, DO

8400 E. Prentice Avenue, Suite 301

Greenwood Village, CO 80111

Phone: (303) 488-0034

Fax: (303) 488-0040

E-Mail: singerdo@aol.com

Website: www.denver-doctor.com

A Natural Balance Wellness Center

Gary E. Foresman, MD

David M. Marquis, DC, CCN
Tod Thoring, ND
260 #A Station Way
Arroyo Grande, CA 93430
Phone: 805-481-3442
FAX: 805-481-3442
Website: www.anaturalbalance.com

John M. Scott DC
Christopher Village Chiropractic
7313 North 49th Street
Longmont, Colorado 80503
Phone: 303-530-3828
E-mail: JMScottDC@yahoo.com

Brandon Lundell DC Dipl Ac
Chiropractic, Acupuncture, Applied Kinesiology, Nutrition
619 Pratt St.
Longmont, Colorado 80501
Phone: 720-771-0402
Fax: 303-776-9272
Email: brandonlundell@juno.com

CONNETICUT

Stephen T. Sinatra, M.D., F.A.C.C.,

New England Heart Center
483 West Middle Tpke,
Manchester, CT 06040
Phone: 860-643-5101
Fax: 860-533-9747
Website: http://drsinatra.com

George Zabrecky, M.D.
The Americas Research & Treatment Center
424a Main Street
Ridgefield, Conneticut 06877
Phone: (203) 438-4762
Fax: (203) 438-4791

Nicholas J. Palermo, D.O., P.C.
49 Erie Street
Manchester, CT 06040
Phone: 860-659-5999
E-Mail: NPal525749@aol.com

DELAWARE

Gertie Hillman, R.N.
Nutrition The Way To Life
412 E. Savannah
Lewes, Delaware 11958
(302) 645-1696
Fax: (302) 645-4940

E-Mail: gerties.nutrition@verizon.net

(R.N. Hillman is a Certified Nutritionist and Herbalist and uses Poly-MVA in her Holistic Nutrition Counseling)

FLORIDA

Leslie Ann Bartlett, D.C.
4505 Chuluota Rd
Orlando, Florida 32820
(407) 568-0909

Martin Dayton, D.O., M.D.
Dayton Medical Office
18600 Collins Avenue
Sunny Isles Beach, Florida 33160
(305) 931-8484
E-Mail: mdayton@the-beach.net
Website: www.daytonmedical.com/

David Minkoff, M.D.
301 Turner Avenue
Clear Water, Florida 33755
(727) 466-6789

George Collins, Nutritional Consultant
Life Extension Nutrition Center

661 N. Orlando Avenue

Maitland, Florida 32751

Phone:1-800-529-1163

Email: geo_lenc@yahoo.com

Judy Blonk, CNC

(Certified Nutrition Consultant, Massage & Colon Therapy)

Natural Health Options

235 E. Nine Mile Road

Pennsacola,, FLA. 32534

Phone: 850-484-0482

Ray Wunderlich, M.D.

Wunderlich Center For Nutritional Medicine

1152 94th Avenue North

St. Peterburg, Florida 33702

Phone: 727-822-3612

Product Information Number 727-577-4344

Email: debbie@wunderlichcenter.com

Website: www.wunderlichcenter.com

Jeffrey Mueller MD

Mueller Institute For Functional Medicine & Research

251 Maitland Ave. Ste. 104

Altamonte Springs, FL 32701

Phone: (407) 332-5703

Fax: (4070 332-5744

E-Mail: Mueller@MuellerInstitute.com

Web Site: www.muellerinstitute.com

Bob Didonato MD
Advanced Medicine
2180 West First Street
Fort Myers, Florida 33901
Phone: (239) 461-0330
Fax: (239) 461-0340
Email: AndreaDidonato@yahoo.com

Tim Blend MD
Anti-Aging/Regenerative Medicine
4216 Cortez Road
Bradenton, FL 34210
941-739-2225
Email: tblend@ihafl.net
Website: http://www.ihafl.com

Frank Maye DOM NMD
Maye Holisitc Med, Inc.
Naturopath, Acupuncture
7800 SW 57th Avenue, Suite 126
Miami, Florida 33143
Phone: 305-668-9555
Email: MayeHolisticMed@aol.com
Website: www.MayeHolisticMed.com

Sharon Perlow, N.D., M.S., ABAAHP
Aventura Longevity Institute, Inc.
18851 NE 29th Ave, Suite 739
Aventura, Florida 33180
Phone: (305) 793-9117
Fax: (305) 907-2435
E-Mail: longevityali@aol.com

GEORGIA

Stephen B. Edelson, M.D.
The Edelson Center For Environmental &
Preventive Medicine
3833 Roswell Road, Suite 110
Atlanta, Georgia 30342
Phone: (404) 841-0088
Fax: (404) 841-6416
Website: www.edelsoncenter.com/

Rhett Bergeron, M.D.
American Wellness Center
(Metabolic Medicine, Cancer, Nutrition and Immune Therapies)
175 Country Club Drive (Atlanta Metro Area)
Stockbridge, Georgia 30281
Phone: (770) 474-8700
E-Mail: RBergeron.MD@worldims.com

Nancy C. Farley, PhD
(Psychologist & Cancer Survivor)
625 Lexington Way
Woodstock, Georgia 30189
Phone: 770-592-8775
E-mail: nfhaven@attbi.com

Michelle M. Fischer, MD
Anti-Aging and Vitality Center of Atlanta
325 Hammond Drive, Suite 204
Sandy Springs, GA 30328
Phone: (404) 255-5583
Fax: (404) 255-5593
E-mail: mmf7@bellsouth.net
Website: www.antiagingandvitality.com
Areas of speciality: Anti-aging, functional and regenerative medicine

---

HAWAII

Tom Yarema, M.D.
Kauai Center For Holistic Research
4504 Kukui Street, Suite 13
Kapaa, Hawaii 96746
Phone: 808-823-0994
Fax: 808-823-0995

IDAHO

Marian English MA NCBMT
600 North Main
P.O. Box 4081
Ketchum, Idaho 83340
Bus-Phone: (208) 727-6975
Email: afreerange@earthlink.net

My Practice: Holistic Health :Practitioner specializing in applied intuition - energy work, massage, counseling, applied kinesiology. also certified gyrotonic and pilates instructor.

ILLINOIS

Janet Fakhouri, N.D., N.C., M.S.
Custom Health, Inc.
10748 South Cook Avenue
Oak Lawn, IL. 60453
708-261-7178

James Corzine DC
Accident & Chronic Pain Center
210 West Market Street
Christopher, Illinois 62822
Phone: 618-724-9200
E-mail: jcorzine@shawneelink.net

Oscar I. Ordonez MD
Belvidere Center For Health & Nutrition
6413 Logan Avenue, Suite 104
Belvidere, Illinois 61008
Phone: (815} 544-3112
Fax: {815) 544-3114
Email: OIOMD1@netzero.com

INDIANA

BODY-N-BALANCE, INC.
Barbara Hunter
LPN, APH, DIHom (Pract.) Board Certified
Homeopathic Practitioner
Biofeedback Stress Testing (EDS)
578 Geiger Drive Suite B Roanoke, Indiana 46783 Phone 260-672-2339 Fax 260-672-8748 E-mail:barbara@bodynbalance.org
Website: www.bodynbalance.org

Marvin Dziabis MD
Health Restoration Clinic
107 W 7th St.
North Manchester, IN 46962
Phone: 260-982-1400
Fax: 260-982-1700
E-mail: Dziabis@aol.com
Website: www.medical-library.net/doctors/health_restoration_clinic/

Arthur Sumrall, M.D.
Longevity Institute of Indiana
9292 North Meridian Street, Suite 300
Indianapolis, Indiana 46260
Phones: 317-924-5655; 317-574-1677
E-mail: info@drsumrall.com
Website: http://www.longevity-inst.com

Oscar I. Ordonez MD
Randolph Health Associates
218 S. Main Street
Parker City, Indiana 47368
Phone: (765) 468-6337
Fax: (765) 287-0161
Email: OIOMD1@netzero.com

I CAN BE HEALTHY LLC
David A. Darbro, MD, Medical Director
9801 Fall Creek Road, #501
Indianapolis, IN 46256
Phone:317-855-7266
Email: drdavid@darbromd.com

KANSAS

John Toth, M.D.
Luke Center For Alternative Medicine

2115 S.W. Tenth Street,
Topeka, Kansas 66604
Phone: 785 232-3330
Fax: 785-232-1874
E-mail: lukecenter@aol.com

Ron Hunninghake MD
Center For the Improvement of Human Functioning
3100 North Hillside Avenue,
Wichita, KS 67219
Phone: (316) 682-3100
Fax: (316) 618-8537
E-mail: docron@brightspot.org
Web Page: www.brightspot.org

MARYLAND

Irwin J. Rosenberg, P.D.
(Doctor of Pharmacy)
Apothecary
5415 Cedar Lane, Suite 102 B
Bethesda, Maryland 20814
Phone: 301-530-4013
E-mail: apoth123@aol.com

Barbara Johnson, R.N.
3605 Southside Avenue
Phoenix, Maryland 21131-173

Office: 410-628-6877

E-Mail: bjohnsonrn@aol.com

Peter G. Marinakis Ac MD
Specialty: Chinese Medicine
Full Circle Healing Arts
645 Ridgely Ave
Annapolis, MD 21401
Business Phone: 410-266=9370
Fax Phone: 410-266-3902
Email: pmarinakis@riva.net
WebSite: www.fullcirclehealingarts.com

My Practice: Full circle healing arts offers an alternative health care

practice offerring western medicine, chinese and western herbs, IV

nutritionals, massage, acupuncture, psychotherapy in the Annapolis, MD area.

MICHIGAN

Linda K. Hegstrand, MD, PhD
Blue Heron Academy of Healing Arts and Sciences
2040 Raybrook SE Suite 104
Grand Rapids, MI 49546
Phone: 616-974-9004
E-Mail: Lhegstrand@aol.com

Steven Margolis, M.D.
(Family Practice Physician)
Alternacare Clinic
37300 Dequindre Road, Suite 201
Sterling Heights, Michigan 48310
Phone: 586-268-0228
Fax: 586-268-7392
E-Mail:Alternacare@hotmail.com

MINNESOTA

Mae Beth Lindstrom, D.C.
Slayton Chiropractic Clinic, P.A.
2002 Broadway
Slayton, Minnesota 56712
(507) 836-8911

Jean O'Hern, N.D.
Nature's Wisdom
2516 Lyndale Avenue South
Minneapolis, Minnesota 55405
Phone: 612-872-4210
E-Mail: johern@usinternet.com

Jeffrey Essen, ND, CEDS
14112 Park Avenue

Burnsville, Minnesota 55337

Phone: (612) 987-4703

E-mail: jessen@mauimail.com

MISSISSIPPI

Dr. Arnold Smith, MD
North Central Mississippi Regional Cancer Center
1401 River Road
Greenwood, MS 38930
Phone: 662-459-7133 Fax: 662-459-7136
Website: http://www.cancernet.com/

MISSOURI

Norman A. Smith, N.M.D., D.C.
Paul A. Campbell, N.M.D.
LifeStyle Wellness Center
307 Main Street, Box 37
Pineville, Missouri 64856
Office-417-223-4103 Fax 417-223-4103
E-Mail: ARCTICUS@aol.com

Wesley Delport, ND
Abundant Health and Wellness

4323 S. National Avenue

Springfield, Mo. 65810

Office-417-890-7400 Toll Free 800-528-7796

E-Mail: abundanthealth@sbcglobal.net

Website: www.getwellnaturally.net

Charles C. Thao, N.M.D., Ph.D.

MEDYCINEX, LLC

2332 W. Woodbury Street

Springfield, MO 65807

Office: 417-886-7184

E-Mail: drcharles@thao.com

Website: www.zoomob.net

NEVADA

James W. Forsythe, M.D., H.M.D.

Cancer Screening and Treatment Center of Nevada

521 Hammill Lane

Reno, NV 89511

Phone: (775) 827-0707

Fax: (775) 827-1006

e-mail: info@drforsythe.com

Web: www.drforsythe.com

Thomas Brumfield, M.D.

Las Vegas Institute of Preventive Medicine
601 S. Rancho Drive, Suite B-16
Las Vegas, Nevada 89106
(702) 380-8470
E-Mail: drbrumfield@lasvegasiopm.com
Website:www.lasvegasiopm.com/index.html

Robert D. Milne, M.D.
Milne Medical Center
2110 Pinto Lane
Las Vegas, Nevada 89106
(702)385-1393
E-Mail: mmc@lvcm.com

Fuller Royal, M.D., H.M.D.
The Nevada Clinic
3663 Pecos-McLeod
Las Vegas, Nevada 89121
Phone: 702-732-1400
E-Mail: FFRoyal@NevadaClinic.com
Website: www.NevadaClinic.com

W. Douglas Brodie MD
6110 Plumas St. Suite B,
Reno, Nevada 89509
(775) 829-1009
(775) 829-9330
E-mail: jorge@drbrodie.com
Website: www.drbrodie.com

Michael Gerber M.D., H.M.D
Gerber Medical Clinic
3670 Grant Drive, Suite 101
Reno, Nevada 89509
Phone 775-826-1900
Fax: 775-826-0578
E-Mail: DrGerber@GerberMedical.com
Website: http://www.gerbermedical.com/

NEW HAMPSHIRE

Jack M. Larmer, ND
A Practice of Natural Health Care Since 1952
P.O. Box 3572
Nashua, New Hampshire 06061-3572
Toll Free: 888-273-3316
Email: JMLarmerND@aol.com
Web Site: http://users.aol.com/jmlarmernd/Naturopathic-Doctor-index.html

---

NEW JERSEY

Hyman Greenfield, M.D.
Center For Progressive Medicine
Century Office Building
216 Haddon Ave., Suite 608

Westmont NJ 08108

Phone: 856-779-8223

Fax: 609-779-7644

E-Mail: hygreen@bigfoot.com

Website: http://earthmed.netreach.net/centprog

Dr. Alfred Hitman, ND, RD
Mind Body Wellness Center

45 Academy Street, Suite 301

Newark, New Jersey 07102

Phone: (973) 242-7271

E-mail: A.HITMAN@att.net

Web Page: http://mindbodywellnesscenter.net

Stuart H. Freedenfeld, MD
Stockton Family Practice

56 South Main St

Stockton, NJ 08559

Phone: 609-397-8585

E-mail: info@stocktonfp.com

Website: http://www.StocktonFP.com

Joel Arcilla MD
Better Living Lifestyle Center

42 Evelyn B. Morine Blvd

Berlin, NJ 08009

Business: (856) 719-6739

Business Fax: (856) 719-1579

E-mail: bllc@comcast.net

Web Page: www.BetterLivingCenter.org

NEW MEXICO

Joseph Breslin, N.D.
Life Medical Group
HC 78, Box 9531
Rancho de Taos, New Mexico 87557
E-Mail: kpettit@newmex.com

Dennis Kramer, Board Certified ND
Board Qualified Thermographic Technician
2308 Camino Vado
Santa Fe, New Mexico 87507
Phone: 505-424-8808
E-mail: biodoc@aol.com

NEW YORK

Richard Ross, M.D.
175 Jericho Turnpike,
Suite 212
Syosset, New York 11791
516-496-7677

Michael B. Schachter, M.D.
Two Executive Blvd., Suite 202

Suffern, New York 10901

(845) 368-4700

E-Mail: office@mbschachter.com

Website: www.mbschachter.com

Dr. John A. Casey, C.C.N.
Flatbush Natural Health Center
142 E. 56th Street

Brooklyn,, New York 11203

Phone: 718-498-5010

E-mail: drjcasey@aol.com

David Borenstein, MD

866 East 29th St.

Brooklyn, NY 11210

Phone: 718-758-1650

Fax: 718-758-1654

E-mail: dboren@pol.net

Website: www.davidborensteinmd.com

NORTH CAROLINA

Bill Crawford ND
Abundant Health Co-operative
1550 E. Main Street

Franklin, North Carolina 28734

Office: 828-524-1100

Home: 828-524-9642

Fax: 828-349-1367

Cell: 828-342-1753

Mailto:BillCrawfordND@verizon.net

(Dr. Crawford's Clinic has staff for Acupuncture and Massage Therapy in addition to Naturopathy.)

Eileen M. Wright, M.D., F.A.C.E.P.

John Wilson, M.D.

Great Smokies Medical Center, P.A.

(Metabolic, Nutritional, Preventive Medicine, Chelation Therapy & Acupuncture)

Asheville Location:

Park Terrace Center, 1312 Patton Ave.

Asheville, North Carolina 28806

Phone: (828)252-9833

Fax: (828)255-8118

E-Mail: greatsmo@aol.com

Statesville Location:

Plaza 21 North, US Route 21,

P.O. Box 6981

Statesville, North Carolina 28687

Phone: (704)876-1617

Fax: (704)876-0640

Rashid A. Buttar, DO, FACAM, FAAPM

Advanced Concepts In Alternative And Preventive Medicine
20721 Torrence Chapel Road, Suite 101 - 102
Cornelius, North Carolina 28031
Phone: 704-895-9355
Fax: 704-895-9357
E-Mail: drbuttarclinic@aol.com
Website: www.drbuttar.com

Joe Carr, N.D.
Wellness Therapies, Browning Plaza 2
4010 Oleander Drive, Suite 10,
Wilmington, North Carolina 28403
Phone: 910-452-4060
E-Mail: joecarr@wellnesstherapies.net
Website: www.wellnesstherapies.net

OHIO

Janis Bell, Ph.D., Dipl. B.N., Bal., NMD
Healing Arts
20090 New Gambier Rd.
Gambier, OH 43022
740-427-2650
E-Mail: drjanisbell@ecr.net

William D. Mitchell, D.O.
Specialist in Internal & Integrative Medicine
Physicians Care Center, Inc.
10034 Brewster Lane
Powell, Ohio 43065
(Greater Columbus Area)
Phone: 614-761-0555
Fax: 614-761-8937
E-Mail: wmitchell@ascinet.com

James LaValle, RPH, N.D., CCN
Living Longer Institute
5400 Kennedy Avenue
Cincinnati, Ohio 45248
Phone: 513-281-3400, Ext 147
Fax: 513-351-3800
E-Mail: jlavelle@proscan.com
Web Page: http://www.livinglonger.com

George Stroia, N.D.
Andrea Stern, N.D.
"Mend Your Body, Inc."
12760 Chillicothe Rd.
Chesterland, Ohio 44026
Phone: 440-729-9695
Fax: 440-729-3580 fax
Email: mendbody@ncweb.com

Ho Young Chung, D.O.
Get Well Center

635 S. Trimble Road

Mansfield, Ohio 44906

Phone: (419) 524-2676

Fax: (419) 524-2692

E-mail: DrHYChung@aol.com

Get Well Center
Theodore Togliatti MD
Steven Mann DO
Insook Chung RN MSN FNP

635 S. Trimble Road

Mansfield, Ohio 44906

Phone: (419) 524-2676

Fax: (419) 524-2692

Email: ChungGWC@aol.com

OKLAHOMA

Dr. Paul Rothwell, M.D.
Wellness and Longevity

7530 NW 23rd Street

Bethany, Oklahoma 73008

Phone: (405)787-8556

Fax: (405) 787-7424

Email: info@wellnessok.com

Website: www.wellnessok.com

Robert L. White, N.D., P.A.
Genesis Medical Research
817 S.W. 89th
Oklahoma City OK 73139
Phone: 405-634-7855
E-mail: gmrs@cox.net

Mary Schrick, N.D.
***Full Circle Health Clinic**
3601 S. Broadway
Edmond OK 73013
Phone: (405) 753-9355
E-mail: maryschrick@sbcglobal.net

***Doorway To Good Health**
Health Food & Supplements
2512 N. Meridian
Oklahoma City, Oklahoma 73120
405-947-2273

Lou Phillips, ND
Carla Phillips, ND
Meridian Avenue Nutrition
1321 N. Meridian Avenue
Oklahoma City, Oklahoma 73107
Phone: 405-943-6000
Toll-free: 800-221-4973
E-mail: :meridianflorist@aol.com

James Hopkins, N.D.
4801 N. Classen Blvd.
Oklahoma City, Ok. 73118
Phone: 405-946-6138
Email: hopkinsdr@earthlink.net

James Hogin DO
James W Hogin Medical Center
937 SW 89th St, Suite #C,
Oklahoma City, OK 73139
Phone: (405) 631-0524
Email: jwhoginmed@coxinet.net

OREGON

Dr. Kenneth Welker, M.D.
Oregon Optimal Health
1200 Executive Parkway, Suite 360
Eugene, OR 97401
Phone: 541-762-1155
Fax: 541-762-1154
Website: www.oregonoptimalhealth.com

PENNSYLVANIA

June Ferrari, N.D., CNC

205 West Street Rd.

Feasterville, Pennsylvania 19053

(215) 364-6505

Greg Maurer, M.S.,C.N.C.,DiHom
Rios Nurtition & Medical Products

35 S. Morton Avenue

Morton PA. 19081 (Philadelphia Area)

Phone: 610-543-1858

E-Mail: mailto:maurer3@hotmail.com

F. Patrick Tierney, ND DC

14 Orchard Rd.

Hummelstown, PA 17036

Phone: (717) 566-7903

Fax: (717) 566-4170

E-mail: drfptierney@hotmail.com

RHODE ISLAND

Zofia Laszewski, M.D.

11 Money Hill Road,

P.O. Box 733

Chepachet, Rode Island 02814

Office Phone: (401) 568-0648

Fax Phone: (401) 568-0649

E-Mail: instzlmd@aol.com

John Curran, M.D., N.D.
Rhode Island Health Aid,
743 Reservior Avenue
Cranston, Rode Island 02910
Phone: 401-946-7602
E-Mail: info@DrCurran.com
Website: www.DrCurran.com

TEXAS

Dee Simmons, Director
Ultimate Living
(For information speak to: Dee's Assistant: Rojene Tadlock)
3402 Oak Grove, Suite 300
Dallas, Texas 75204
Phone: 214-220-1240
E-Mail: ultimateliving@hawkpci.net
Web Page: www.ultimateliving.com

Stephen L. Duncan, LTH, RMT
Liscensed Theocentric Healer-Registered Massage Therapist
Body Works Holistic Spa
9205 Skillman Street, Suite 115
Dallas, Texas 75243
Phone: 877--891-5651

E-Mail: healingzone@aol.com

Web Page: www.holisticbodyworker.com

Loretta Lanphier ND CCN HHP
Oasis Advanced Wellness
9842 Pinehurst Drive

Baytown TX 77521

Phone: (281) 303-0707

Fax: (281) 573-4556

Email: staff@oasisadvancedwellness.com

Website: www.drlorettalanphier.byregion.net

Kathleen Jackson, N.M.D., RPH
Optimal Health Hub
2800 Broadway C-715

Pearland, Tx 77581

Phone: 281-705-2679

Email: askkathy@gmail.com

Website: www.optimalhealthhub.com

UTAH

Jeanne Wallace, PhD, CNC
Nutritional Solutions
1697 East 3450 North

North Logan, Utah 84341

Phone: (435) 563-0053

Fax: (435) 563-0052

E-Mail: nutritionalsolutions@comcast.net

website: www.nutritional-solutions.net

(Dr. Wallace has her Ph.D in Nutrition and is a specialist in treating brain tumors with Integrative Holistic Nutrition including Poly-MVA.)

Sherman Johnson, M.D.
Young Life Research Clinic
1275 North 750 West,

Springville, Utah 84663

Phone: 801-489-8650

E-Mail: shjohnson@youngliving.com

Cordell E. Logan ND
Total Health Institute
385 W 600 N

Lindon Utah 84042

801-796-8111

E-mail: cordell@agclinic.com

Website http://www.agclinic.com

VERMONT

Julian Jonas, CCH, Lic. Ac.
Center for Homeopathy of Southern Vermont

220 Western Avenue
Brattleboro, VT 05301
Office: 802-254-2928

Fax: 802-246-4080
jjjonas@sover.net
www.centerforhomeopathy.com

VIRGINIA

Manjit Bajwa MD
Comprehensive Medical Center
6391 Little River Turnpike
Alexandria, VA 22312
Office: 703-941-3606
Fax: 703-658-6415
Email: drbajwa11@netzero.net
Website: http://altmedsite.com/index.html

Practice: Chelation, Mercury & Metal Detox, Hyperbaric Oxygen Chamber, Bioidentical hormones & Anti-aging, Chronic fatigue, Hypothyroidism, adjunctive treatments of Cancer & chronic diseases with Exercise diet, detoxification

Robert Hutt, M.D.
Alternative Care
550 Broadview Ave., Suite 202

Warrenton, VA. 20186

Phone: 540-450-2763

Email: hutt@infi.net

Mitchell A. Fleisher, M.D., D.Ht., F.A.A.F.P.
Homeopathic Family Medicine & Nutritional Therapy

Rockfish Center, Suite 1, S.R. 664, P.O. Box 303

Nellysford, Virginia U.S.A. 22958-0303

Phone: (434) 361-1896

Fax: (434) 361-1928

E-mail: info@alternativemedcare.com

Website: www.alternativemedcare.com

WASHINGTON

Dr. Elizabeth Hesse DC CCN
Experience Health!

502 S. Sullivan Rd. Suite 106

Veradale WA 99037

509-927-7155

E-Mail: drhessedc@aol.com

WebSite: www.experiencehealthcenter.com

Ella Hill, R.N., LMHC
(Counsels patients for emotional, medical and nutritional needs)
EMH Counseling Center

2101 Fourth Avenue, Suite 1370
Seattle, Washington 98121
Phone: 206-441-0926
E-Mail: ella1370@aol.com
Website: www.ellamhill.com

Kathryn L. Poleson, DMD
(General Dentist)
Vancouver, WA
(Dr. Poleson highly endorses Poly-MVA and publicly recommends it to her professional colleagues, but does not use it in her practice.)
E-Mail: WAGDEditor@juno.com
Areas of Specialty: Preventive and Restorative Dentistry
"I feel fortunate in having met Dr. Garnett. His work and its results are incredible. It is thrilling to speak to a woman patient who chose not to have a mastectomy and now is cancer free - and has been for three years - because she searched for a healthy answer and found Poly-MVA."

Robert Jangaard, ND
1657 E. Layton Road
Freeland, WA 98249
Phone: (360) 331-6470
E-mail: jangaard@whidbey.com

WYOMING

Rebecca Painter, M.D., P.C.
Internal Medicine
201 West Lakeway, Suite 300
Gillette, Wyoming 82718
Phone: 307-682-0330
Fax: 307-686-8118
Toll Free: 1-800-553-3100
E-Mail: drpainter@vcn.com

Jonathan W. Singer, DO
1401 Airport Parkway, Suite 150,
Cheyenne, WY 82001
Phone: (307) 635-4362
E-Mail: singerdo@aol.com

International Practitioners

ARUBA, DUTCH WEST INDIES

Carlos Viana, PhD, OMD, CAd, FACACN
Viana Natural Healing Center
Kibaima 7, Aruba, Dutch West Indies
Telephone: (297) 85 1270

Fax: (297) 85 4789

E-Mail: drcarlos52@hotmail.com

Jose' V. A. Humphreys NMD DNM
Optimum Health Clinic
P.O. Box W1280
Belvedere Estate
St. John's
Antigua, West Indies
drjhumphreys@gmail.com

BAHAMAS

Dr. Sir Kevin C. King N.D M.D.(M.A.) F.R.C.P.
The Natural Health Clinic
#4 Lucayan Plaza
Coral Road
Freeport, Grand Bahama
Bahamas
1-242-373-8102
1-242-373-1052-fax
E-Mail: sir_kevinking@hotmail.com

CANADA

Jim Chan ND

3331-No. 3 Road

Richmond, BC

Canada V6X 2B6

Phone: (604)273-4372

E-Mail: Info@drjimchan.com

Website: www.drjimchan.com

Jose D'Costa Reis, N.D.

108 Yorkville Avenue, Suite #4

Toronto, Ontario

CANADA M5R-1B9

(416) 968-0300

(416) 968-0201

Fateh Srajeldin, N.D.

5468 Dundas St. West # 101

Etobicoke, Ontario

CANADA M9B-6E3

Phone: (416) 207-0207

Fax: (416) 207-0272

E-Mail: doctor@doctorallergies.com

Website: www.doctorallergies.com/index.html

Howard Turner, M.D.

19 Cours Le Royer West, Suite 106

Montreal, Quebec

Canada H2Y 1W4

Phone: 514-931-2021 Fax: 514-285-9231

E-Mail: DrHTurner@hotmail.com

Dr. Ahmad Nasri
Nasri Chelation & Integrative Medicine
730 Essa Road
Barrie, Ontario,
Canada L4N 9E9
Phone: 705-735-2354
Toronto Office:
Phone: 647-293-5363
E-Mail: nasrichelation@rogers.com
Website: www.nasrichelation.com

Veronica Wolff, BSc, RNCP
(Registered Holistic Nutritionist with specialty in Darkfield Blood Analysis)
2055 Parklane Crescent
Burlington, Ontario,
Canada L7M 3V6
Phone: 905-336-4040
E-Mail: vwolff1@cogeco.ca

John H. Biggs, RNC, BSc
(Registered Nutrition Consultant)
Optimum Health Choices
11646-104 Avenue
Edmonton, Alberta,
Canada T5K 2T7
Phone: 780-439-5748
E-Mail: opti1@oanet.com

Website: www.optimumhealthvitamins.com

Katherine Willow, N.D.
4596 Carp Road
Carp, Ontario, K0A 1L0
Canada K0A 1L0
Phone: 613-839-1179
Fax: 613-839-3909
E-mail: katherine@echelon.ca

Arun Dosaj, M.D.
AntiAging and Wellness Clinic
41 St. Lawrence St. E.,
Box 750
Madoc, Ontario
Canada K0K 2K0
Phone: 613-473-5222
Fax: 613-473-4272
E-Mail: drdosaj@hotmail.com
Website: www.mydoc.ca

William Russell ND
Semiahmoo Wellness Center
#102 15585 24th Ave.
Surrey, British Columbia
Canada V4A 2J4
Business Phone: (604) 535-4003
Fax Phone: (604) 535-4201
Email: raddysh@telus.net

WebSite: www.askdoctorbill.com

My Practice: Whole body approach to health. Treat a wide variety of chronic conditions.Use IV chelation therapies.

DOMINICAN REPUBLIC

George Zabrecky, M.D.
The Americas Research & Treatment Center
El Vergel #45 Ortega y Gasset
Santa Domingo, Dominican Republic
Phone: (809) 472-1238
Fax: (809) 567-8386

GERMANY

Freidrich R. Douwes, M.D.
Klinik St. Georg
Rosenheimer Strabe 6-8
83043 Bad Aibling, Germany
Phone: 011-49-8061-398-428
Fax: 011-49-8061-398-454
E-Mail: : info@klinik-st-georg.de
Website: www.klinik-st-georg.de

ITALY

Fiamma Ferraro MD
Via Paganella 7A
00135 Roma, Italy
Business Tel. (+39)0635500018
Cell Tel. (+39)3403754383
Email: fiafer@yahoo.com
Website: www.geocities.com/fiafer

JAPAN

Andrew Wong MD PhD
Roppongi Dr. Andy`s Clinic of Plastic & Cosmetic Surgery and Age Management Medicine
6/7 F Roppongi Shimada Bldg.,
4-8-7, Roppongi, Minato-ku
Tokyo, Japan 106-0032
Phone: 81-3-3401-0720
Fax: 81-3-3401-0704
E-mail: andy@drandy.com
Web Page: www.drandy.com

LEBANON

Tony Georges Lichaa, M.D.

(Specialist in Internal Medicine & Cardiology Trained at the Montreal Heart Institute, American Board of Chelation Therapy)

Beirut Location:

The Anti-Aging and Life Rejuvenating Medical Center
Verdun Plaza One, 2nd Floor
Beirut, Lebanon
Phone: 961 3 25 49 45
EMail: tlichaa@inco.com.lb

Jounieh Location:

The Medical Center For Prevention And The Treatment Of Diseases
P.O. Box 245
Jounieh, Lebanon
Phone: 961 9 911 875
FAX 961 9 914 195
EMail: tlichaa@inco.com.lb

MEXICO

Mexico City
Amarc Mexico
Phone # 85-96-0881 55-74-8183
Fax # 85-96-0880

Mexico D.F.,Guerrero,Tabasco,Toluca
Dr.Leticia Perez:
Consultorio 57966515
Cel. (044)26765474
E-mail: joe112@hotmail.com

Jose Luis Rodriguez
consultorio 57966515
Cel. (044)19225858
E-Mail: joe112@hotmail.com

Mexico, D.F.
Dr. Luis Ramirez- Consultorio 56495987
Cel. (044)25431183 - (044) 50426961
Tulancingo Hidalgo, Puebla

Dr. Vargas
Consultorio 77552434
Fax 77555818

Monterrey
Dr. Braulio Ayala
Consultorio 83005267
Casa: 83470943

Monterrey
Braulio Ayala
Phone# 83005267
Fax # 83470943

Sonora:

Jose A. Miranda

Phone# 33302177

Hermosillo, Sonora

Zaida Pax

Consultorio 62120330

Fax 62170945

Jose A. Miranda

Consultorio (333) 02177

PHILIPPINE ISLANDS

GREEN & GOLD INTL EXPORTS

Manny Kiok

RM 307 SOLMAC BLDG

84 DAPITAN ST

1114 QUEZON CITY, PHILIPPINES

Phone: 011-632-415-8714

Jaime E. Dy-Liacco, D.M.M.

29 Mangyan Road

1108 Quezon City

Philippines

Phone: 011-632-924-2487, and 011-929-6670

Fax: 011-632-929-9173

E-Mail: mito@pacific.net.ph

Carmencita R. Yap, M.D.
Twin Hearts Holistic Center
2 Panay Avenue
Quezon City, Philippines
Phone: 011-632-373-2141, and 011-632-411-8450
Fax: 011-632-371-9855
E-Mail: pcam95@yahoo.com

What is the Survival Outlook with Polycythemia Vera?

At present, using a **rational approach** to therapy tailored to the individual patient, the survival with PV is commonly 10 - 20 years.

Most patients **succumb** to other **co-morbid diseases** that come with aging, such as heart disease or cancers.

Without any treatment, the **survival** after diagnosis averages just **2 years**, and so it is crucial to get appropriate therapy and be carefully monitored by a specialized physician.

If proper care is attended to the disease, there is **little reason** for the average patient with PV to have a **reduced life expectancy** owing to PV itself.

Thus, there is more hope today than ever for PV patients to have a normal lifespan.

Made in the USA
Monee, IL
26 May 2021